DRUGS DID THIS

STORIES OF SUBSTANCE ABUSE
IN THE CENTER OF THE TAR HEEL STATE:
PEOPLE WHO DIED,
PEOPLE WHO HAVE BATTLED,
AND PEOPLE WHO ARE BATTLING STILL

BY CHIP WOMICK
PHOTOGRAPHS BY PAUL CHURCH

PeaceLight Press

The information in this book is true and complete to the best of our
knowledge. It is offered without guarantee on the part of the author or
PeaceLight Press. The author and PeaceLight Press disclaim all liability
in connection with the use of this book.

ISBN: 978-0-9971661-4-9

Cover design by Amber Mabe
Back cover photo by Paul Church/Courtesy The Courier-Tribune
www.peacelightpress.com
Printed in the United States of America

For all those touched by substance abuse:
Users, those in recovery,
and the people who love them.
And for the individuals
who bared heart and soul to share these stories.

CONTENTS

PREFACE

This book was conceived after I heard heart-wrenching stories during a candlelight vigil in front of the Randolph County Courthouse in Asheboro in the summer of 2018. The speakers, many of them in tears, were family members of someone who had died from overdose, people who had overcome the demon of substance abuse themselves, and people with loved ones still enslaved by their addictions.

The event was sponsored by the Community Hope Alliance, a growing grassroots organization incorporated in December 2017, committed to providing resources and promoting substance use education, awareness, prevention and safety.

The book has two purposes: to raise money for the multi-pronged mission of the Community Hope Alliance (every penny of proceeds from sales will go to the organization) and to raise awareness of the toll drugs are taking on individuals, their families, and, in fact, on every single person in Randolph County.

* * *

Like cities, counties, and states across the nation, Randolph County faces a challenge in the battle against addiction and overdose deaths, which claimed the lives of more than 72,000 people in the United States in 2017.

The Randolph County Opioid and Drug Community Collaborative was formed to monitor overdose activity and to establish and mobilize collaborative partnerships. The first meeting was held in February 2017. Meetings are open to anyone. Regular attendees include law enforcement personnel, school officials, health care providers and a range of other community members who have an interest in the drug crisis or who provide services to help combat it.

Randolph County Emergency Services began tracking overdose figures – based on reports from first responders – in April of 2017.

◊ April 1-Dec. 31, 2017, there were 194 suspected overdoses and 27 overdose deaths in Randolph County.

◊ In 2018, there were 448 suspected overdoses and 37 overdose deaths.

◊ In the first eight months of 2019, there were 371 suspected overdoses and 27 overdose deaths.

* * *

My drug of choice was alcohol.

I was smitten in high school, the first time I ever drank. As the booze snaked through my bloodstream, I felt a literal rush of warmth that may as well have been radioactive. I grew to love that feeling as my body and mind eased into total relaxation, and my natural shyness melted away.

I drank too much, every time I drank. Night after night, in the early years, I often found myself the last man standing at a party, surrounded by people who had passed out. Most people, of course, had long since had the good sense to stop drinking and go to bed or to go home. The governors that kicked in for those people – whether they were mental, physiological, emotional, or spiritual brakes – I never had them.

I was a fairly well-functioning alcoholic for decades. Which is not really saying a lot. I held down jobs and was a good worker, but I do not care to survey – and certainly do not remember much of – the broken landscape of poor personal interactions that appeared more frequently as the years passed.

Eventually, I kicked my addiction before it killed me, or I killed anyone else. Some struggle mightily, and some never succeed in putting down the bottle, but as best I can tell, the beast of alcohol addiction pales in comparison to the beast of opioid addiction.

When I was growing up in the late 1960s and early 1970s, at least as far as I knew then, heroin was confined to big cities far, far away from my small Southern hometown.

Nearly pure heroin readily available for less than the price of a pack of cigarettes and fentanyl, a synthetic opioid that is 50-100 times more powerful than morphine, were addiction nightmares of the future.

No one expects to get hooked on drugs. Yet, in 2017, the worst year ever for drug overdose deaths in the United States, more than 70,000 people died.

My drug of choice was alcohol. Had I been born a few decades later, might opioids have entered the picture? I do not know.

Chip Womick
September 11, 2019

WHERE THERE IS UNITY

Seeing people, not addicts
Mother/daughter promote harm reduction in Randolph

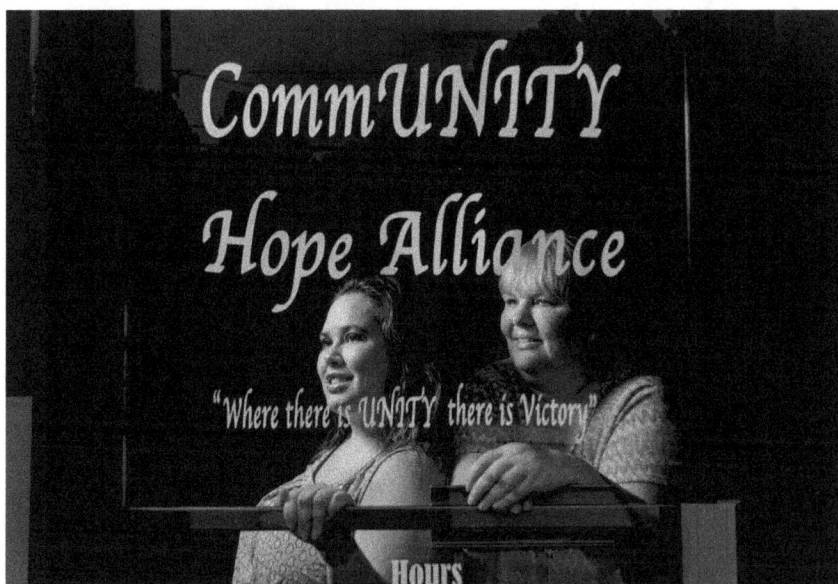

PERSONAL STRUGGLES, PUBLIC SERVICE – Kelly Link, right, and her oldest daughter, Ashley Hedrick, founded the Community Hope Alliance in December 2017. They took action after watching Brett Link (Kelly's son, Ashley's brother) wrestle with substance abuse. (Photograph by Paul Church/The Courier-Tribune)

A few years ago, Kelly Murcin Link was worn out, depressed, and living a nightmare.

When her son, Brett, was using drugs, there was a repeating cycle of lying, stealing, anger, overdose, denial, and incarceration.

She had tried pleading.

She had tried yelling.

She had refused to bail him out of jail, thinking that the reality of being behind bars would get his attention. She had kicked him out of the house, hoping he would come to his senses, and the family could find some peace.

She tossed and turned at night, wondering when the phone would ring with news that he had died from an overdose.

3

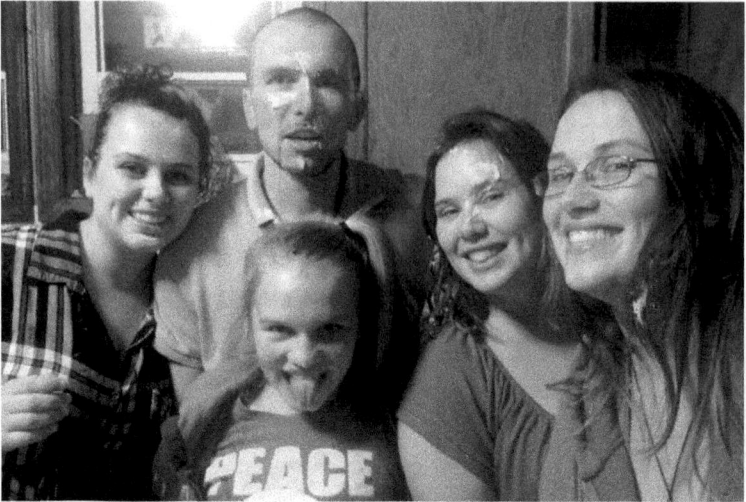

BRETT'S BIRTHDAY – Brett Link poses with his daughter, Felicity (front and center) and his sisters, left to right, Danielle Link, Ashley Hedrick, and Cassie Link at a party to celebrate his birthday. A good time was had by all: Note cake icing on their faces. (Contributed photo)

One sleepless night in 2017, she got out of bed, went to her computer, and began combing the Internet for something.

Answers. Hope. Anything.

It did not take her long to find local groups whose work addressed substance abuse in differing ways. The Greensboro-based Urban Survivors Union was one of them. Soon she had arranged an appointment to meet with Louise Vincent, the organization's executive director.

Link says the first five minutes of conversation with Vincent changed her life. Vincent did not talk about drug users as addicts. She talked about them as people.

"She said when you treat them with a little compassion and love and understanding and meet them where they're at and try to have a conversation with love and compassion, it makes a big difference."

Link left the meeting with a new perspective.

"I was belittling my son and not understanding and not having compassion," she said. "Of course, I loved him, but I was helping him in no way. I was yelling at him and giving him ultimatums, and it was not working."

Back home, she tried a new approach with Brett.

"I've just met an amazing woman," she told him, "and I'm about to do something I never thought that I would do. I want you to stay alive.'"

She gave him clean needles and Narcan and explained how to use the medication that can reverse an opioid overdose.

"He actually opened up," Link said. "He was so happy to have that conversation with me and for me to be open to listen to him and treat him as a person and not as the addict I couldn't stand before.

"He said, 'You will never understand 100 percent, but taking the time to try to understand makes a big difference.'"

Unity, victory

Soon Link was distributing syringes and Narcan (supplied by the Urban Survivors Union) through her son and his friends in Randolph County.

In October 2017, the fledgling effort began operating independently as a state-certified syringe exchange program under the name Asheboro Alliance & Risk Prevention. In the early days, a handful of group participants met regularly at a Randleman fast-food restaurant.

In December 2017, Link and Ashley Hedrick, one of Link's three daughters, registered the group as a North Carolina nonprofit under a new name: Community Hope Alliance (CHA).

"'Unity' is part of the word 'community,'" Link said. "It's all about unity. The 'hope' – we're hoping to change the projection of this epidemic."

The organization's motto is, "Where there is unity, there is victory."

The syringe exchange is the cornerstone of CHA work. "The syringe exchange is keeping people safe," Hedrick said. "We give out supplies, so they don't spread disease and infection."

An August 2019 report from the Centers for Disease Control and Prevention – a federal agency whose goal is to improve public health – said users of syringe services programs were three times more likely to stop injecting drugs.

Hedrick's has a simple take on why syringe exchange programs lead to better outcomes: "It's because somebody gives a crap."

Some participants call Link "Mama."

"I guess they just know they can talk to her," Hedrick said. "They know she's not going to judge them."

"They talk to me and open up," Link said. "They call, or they text, or they message all hours of the night. They're always thanking me, always telling me what a blessing I am."

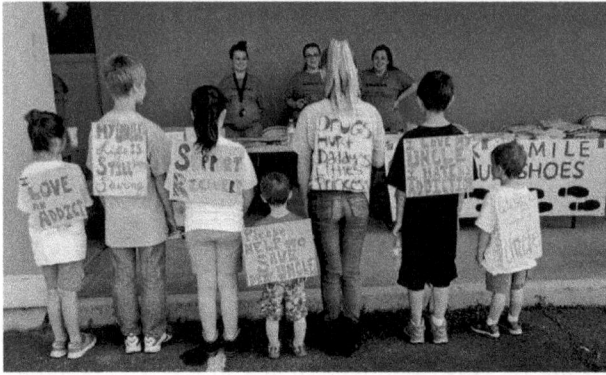

WALKING FOR UNCLE BRETT (AND DAD) – Brett Link's nieces, nephews, and daughter (third from right) wear signs for the first-ever Walk a Mile in Our Shoes event hosted by the Community Hope Alliance in 2018. (Contributed photograph)

She laments that she can do little beyond suggesting resources to contact – and which ones to call first – for those who want to seek treatment.

Injury, pain pills

The starting point in Brett's battle with addiction was a workplace injury when he was 19. He and another fellow were working on scaffolding when something broke. They fell and Brett's 200-pound co-worker landed on top of him, breaking several vertebrae.

Brett was in the hospital for a week, where doctors prescribed OxyContin for the pain, Link said. "It was no time before he was taking more than he should. He quickly became addicted to it. We know several people whose children have had the same experience."

Later, when Brett said he needed more pills before he was due for a refill, he always had a ready excuse, such as saying that he had lost pills down the sink by accident. Before long, he was crushing the pills and snorting the powder, which gets the drug to the bloodstream faster and leads to more intense highs.

At first, his family did not know there was a problem. When they realized something was amiss, they confronted Brett. He admitted what he had been doing and changed his ways. At least that's what they thought.

Soon Brett was drinking too much alcohol, mostly beer, to the point of passing out at night. Then his family discovered that he had replaced prescription pills with cocaine.

This time, they had what Link calls "a real intervention." Brett agreed to enter an inpatient treatment facility in Lexington. Later, they found out that he had sneaked out on the last day of rehab and gone to a bar to drink.

That was two years after the accident. Things went downhill from there.

More pills, prison

A low point came on a snowy winter day when Brett fell, jumped, or was pushed – he later said he did not remember what happened – from a second-floor balcony at an Asheboro motel.

Brett fractured a vertebrae and shattered bones in a foot and wrist in the fall. He needed surgery. Doctors prescribed more pain pills.

"He was 'gone' after that," Link said. "I guarantee he was in pain – and is still in pain. He still walks with a limp."

When Brett wound up in jail for driving without a license, a fellow inmate told him he was "doing" the pills "wrong." The best high, he explained, came not from snorting the powder, but from shooting it up.

Eventually the pipeline of pills Brett could get by prescription dried up. Buying them on the street was expensive, and he started stealing from stores to support his habit.

Brett's family did not know he was injecting drugs until he overdosed. When they arrived at the hospital, he was on a breathing tube, but afterward Brett denied that he had overdosed, and the downward spiral continued. The next time he wound up in the hospital he had a blood infection from using dirty needles.

Then his crimes began to catch up with him, and he served two stints in prison, once for a little less than a year, once for a little more than a year.

"Each time he got out," Link said, "he was clean for a good amount of time."

The last time he relapsed into drug use, Brett tried heroin, and eventually landed in prison again. That's where he has been since March 2018 on convictions for a variety of charges, including conspiracy to sell a Schedule II controlled substance and felony breaking and entering. His current release date is August of 2020, but he has future court dates on pending charges in Randolph and other counties.

The 'goodness' hides

Hedrick said her brother has a quick temper but a heart of gold.

"Even when my brother was the worst in his life, if he was standing in line, he would pay for the little old lady's stuff in line behind him. I know my brother, and I know his heart. He has a good heart, but not when he's on drugs. The goodness in him hides when he's on drugs."

Brett has told his family things about his drug use that surprised them – and that may surprise many people.

Most of the time he used drugs he was trying to avoid the incapacitating sickness that comes with drug withdrawal.

It's even hard to stay clean while incarcerated because drugs are so easy to get behind bars.

And, when he used, he did not really think about overdosing. All he could think about was the blessed relief he would feel when the drugs coursed through his veins.

* * *

What Brett says ...

Note: The following is edited and condensed from answers to questions Kelly Link sent to her son, Brett Link, who is currently serving a sentence in Alexander Correctional Institution in Taylorsville, N. C., for convictions for selling Schedule II controlled substances and felony breaking and entering, among other charges. His current release date is June 14, 2020.

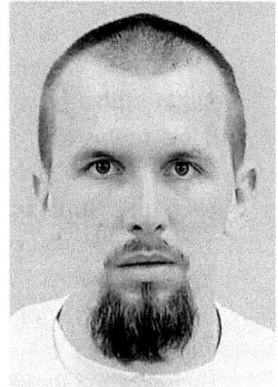

Brett Link

I think I was 8 or 9 years old when I stole one of my dad's weed roaches, but it didn't taste like it smells, and I didn't know that it got you high. It kinda scared me, so I didn't smoke it again until I was like 11-12.

I don't remember the first time I drank, but I remember the first time I got way too drunk. I was about 13. We lived down a long driveway, and I think my mom found me drunk, passed out in the middle of the driveway, on her way home from work. (Moonshine) The first time I used cocaine I was around 15.

I smoked weed regularly from about 14 years old. I started working at Wendy's at 16 and was able to buy my own. I did do cocaine here and there but didn't really get hooked on cocaine until I was about 19.

Hooked on crack

I remember the moment I got hooked. I was at my dad's house alone. I had been upset about a recent break-up for a few days. This guy knocked on the door and wanted a ride. I took him to a house. He went in and came out. A few miles down the road he pulled a pipe out and took a hit of crack. He kept asking if I wanted a hit. I kept saying, "No." I had never smoked it before.

We were coming through a little dirt road. There was a spot where you could pull off the road. He said we could pull off and

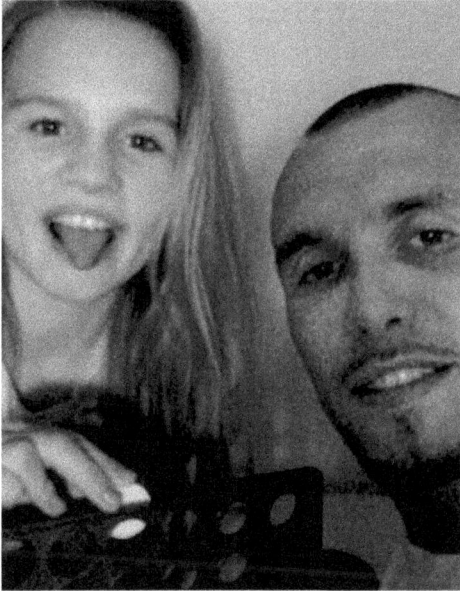

Brett Link and his daughter, Felicity

no one would see us, and I could hit it, and no one would know.

I pulled over and hit it. I dropped him off and went home. But all I could think about was taking a bigger hit. So, the next day I took a bigger hit and slowly went downhill from there.

I didn't like the come down from crack, so I would drink a lot of alcohol really fast and pass out, so I became an alcoholic really fast. My best friend at the time, his mom was a really big coke dealer, so we would get it really cheap. A lot of times for free. Then when it ran out, we would get drunk and call all our friends and party till we passed out.

We literally partied every single day for a few months. We

9

would get high on cocaine and get really quiet and paranoid, and then get drunk and loud and have a blast. We would look at each other and be like, "Why the hell do we do the cocaine and get all paranoid and looking stupid when we can just get drunk and have a blast?"

So, it got to the point where I would wake up and start drinking and party throughout the day. For months I was going into a grocery store and walking out with 6-8 cases of beer in a buggy.

One day I woke up at my dad's house hungover, no money, no ride, no alcohol to drink, and no job. And the worst of all – no family. A couple months before I was with my daughter's mom. We had our own place with the kids. But I got sick of hiding the partying; one day I went home and picked an argument just to get her to move back in with her parents, so I could have the house to myself to party.

That day I woke up at my dad's I had enough. I called my mom and told her I wanted/needed help, and three days later I went to rehab at The Path of Hope in Lexington for 28 days. It is actually a good place. I never quit drinking for good, but I never let myself get like that again or get hooked on crack again.

I think it was about three weeks to a month after I got out of The Path of Hope, I don't know why, but I threw a party at a motel. At the end of the night everyone was gone. I was drunk and somehow fell over the railing two-and-a-half stories up. I shattered my heel and broke my arm and wrist. They gave me prescriptions for oxycodone and 120 Dilaudid.

I didn't know nothing about pills. I actually didn't like pain pills because a couple years before that I broke my back and they gave me Percocet. I drank with them and got really sick. But now I needed these. Someone told me that I could snort them, so I snorted a couple, and I was out of my wheelchair walking around on my cast. Absolutely no pain at all. They had to change my cast because I walked a hole in it.

Three days after they gave me the scripts all 210 pills were gone. I called the doctor and told him I peed in the bed and the pills got wet. He wrote me more scripts. Three or four days later they were gone again. I called and told him someone stole them. He wrote me another two scripts. So, 10-12 days after the first prescriptions, 630 pills were gone. I sold some and gave some away, but I did most of them.

I knew I couldn't call him back again. About three days later, I was so dopesick I wanted to kill myself, so they admitted me to a mental hospital for about a week.

Unbelievably, that wasn't even what got me hooked on opiates.

Little blue pill

About a month after I got out of the mental hospital, they put me in a walking boot. I had not done drugs or drank anything since I been out. I was able to walk, so went to get drunk. The next day my foot hurt so bad I didn't do that again.

About two months later, I finally was out of the walking boot and got a job at a furniture factory. The first day someone that I know saw me limping and saw that I was in pain, so she gave me a little blue pill; she told me to go snort it. It took all the pain away and gave me energy. It was a 10-mg. hydrocodone.

That's where it started. That one hydrocodone turned into one a day, two a day, five a day, to five Percocets a day, to a couple roxys, to five roxys a day, to one 80-mg. oxycodone a day, to 8-10 80-mg. oxycodones a day, to one year in prison.

I got out of prison, got a job, and started all over, but this time I'm shooting up. I went back to prison for eight months. When I got out, I surrounded myself with good people and stayed clean for over a year.

Then I was doing Opanas (oxymorphone) and wound up in prison for four months. I stayed clean for about four months. Then I was heroin and landed back in prison for over two years. I'm 17 months in on this bid now. And I'm doing really good.

Friends lost

I've lost four friends due to drugs in one way or another: Chris Voncannon, Ben Voncannon, Derek Church and Megan Worley. Those were the nicest, caring friends I ever had. Those were all my best friends at one time. I want to add Brittany Boone. She was the sweetest girl I knew. (The Good Die Young!!)

I have never overdosed. I might have done too much a few times and nodded over. I could never trust anyone to save me if I OD'ed, but everyone knew I would save them, so they would try it first, and then I would know how much to do.

I have saved someone 40-50 times with Narcan; I used 12 in one night one time. I saved the same person 4-5 times. It blew my mind they would come back, and I would have to yell at them because they immediately wanted to get high again after they just died.

Staying clean

I am in the most focused and best state of mind I have been in since I started opiates over 10 years ago. It takes quite a while for an opiate addict's brain to come back to normal after they stop using. Mine ain't fully back normal, but it's definitely a lot better than it has been. I don't feel stupid anymore.

You can get whatever kind of drug you want you can get at any time in prison, even if you don't have money; they will still give it to you. You just tell them when you're going to pay. If you don't pay, you get stabbed or cut up.

I have been to treatment before, and I want treatment, but I don't want to be around other addicts. I have not maintained my sobriety in the past because, honestly, I didn't want it. At first, I want to stay clean but then I get sick of having to deal with everything that comes with dealing with life.

But I'm not doing drugs. I'm not smoking. I'm not even taking any meds. My plan to stay clean is to take it one day at a time; stay focused; and, most important, stay away from anyone doing drugs.

Best day of my life

The best day of my life was the day my daughter, Felicity, was born. She is 13. My biggest regret is not being the father I should or could have been.

She says her biggest fear is becoming addicted to drugs. My advice to her is that when (not if) one of her friends comes up to her with drugs and tries to get her to do it, no matter how good a friend they are, or how long they've been friends, or whatever, remember that fear. If you don't say no, I promise it will be the biggest mistake of your life.

You are doing a great job, Felicity. I am really proud of

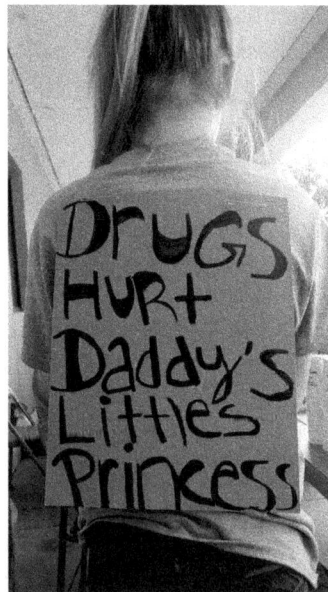

DRUGS HURT DADDY'S PRINCESS – Brett's daughter, Felicity, wears a sign during a march sponsored by the Community Hope Alliance. (Contributed photograph)

you. Be a leader, not a follower. The next 10 years of your life are the most important of your life. All you got to do is stay in school, stay out of trouble, and off drugs, and you can have and be whatever you want.

The future?

I don't know where I will be in five years. I've got pending charges. I could still be in prison, but hopefully not. I would like to talk to kids at schools about drugs. Maybe move to another state out west. Hopefully, Felicity is living with me.

I don't know where I will be in 10 years either. I don't really have a plan. I know I probably should. I would like to own my own business and have a nice, jacked-up truck. And I really want to make up lost time with Felicity. But I can tell you where I won't be in 10 years: Locked up.

Harm reduction is a way of preventing disease and promoting health that 'meets people where they are' rather than making judgments about where they should be in terms of their personal health and lifestyle.

A place of respite
CHA office offers supplies, education, and people who care

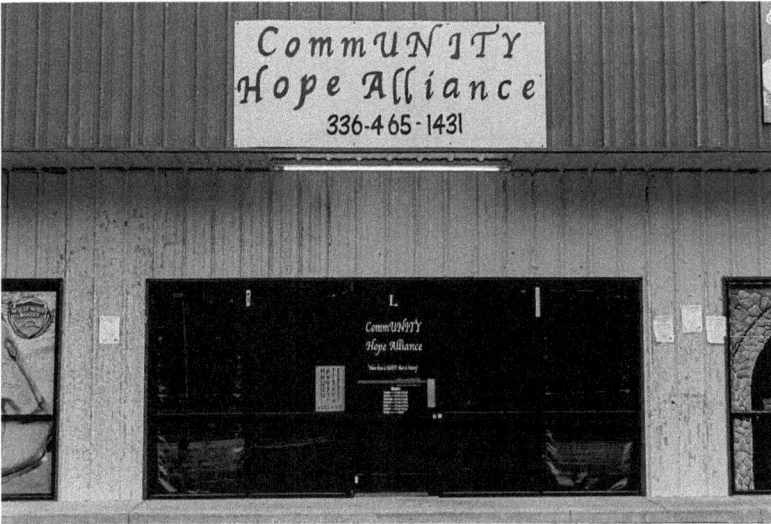

OPEN-DOOR POLICY – The Community Hope Alliance office at 1406 N. Fayetteville St., Unit L, in Asheboro has plush sofas for relaxing; toys, games, and books for children; and a wall on which visitors can draw or write. (Photograph by Paul Church/Courtesy The Courier-Tribune)

The Community Hope Alliance (CHA) services include harm reduction, mobile syringe exchange, naloxone distribution, drug user support and resources, family support and resources, community education, and several public awareness events each year:

◊   Unity Dinner (March)
◊   Walk a Mile in Our Shoes (June)
◊   End Overdose Vigil (August)

According to the North Carolina Harm Reduction Coalition (www.nchrc.org), harm reduction is a way of preventing disease and promoting health that "meets people where they are" rather than making judgments about where they should be in terms of their personal health and lifestyle. Accepting that not everyone is ready or able to stop risky or illegal behavior, harm

15

reduction focuses on promoting scientifically proven ways of mitigating health risks associated with drug use and other high risk behaviors, including condom distribution, access to sterile syringes, medications for opioid dependence such as methadone and buprenorphine, and overdose prevention.

The Community Hope Alliance has distributed more than 75,000 syringes and more than 3,000 naloxone kits. Last year, there were 263 reported overdose reversals using kits the organization distributed.

The log of syringe exchange participants from the early days tops 200 and includes 168 in the past year. Not all are active drug users. Some pick up needles for a loved one. A few, including individuals who need insulin injections, get needles for medical use.

In July 2019, the nonprofit organization opened an office at 1406 N. Fayetteville St., Unit L, in Asheboro. The hours of operation are 6-9 p.m. Monday-Saturday.

It's a place of respite with an open-door policy there are plush sofas for relaxing; toys, games, and books for children; and a wall which visitors can decorate or write a message with colored chalk.

Major funding for 2019 was provided via grants from the Randolph Health Community Foundation and the North Carolina Department of Health and Human Services. CHA also receives cash donations and raises money through the sale of T-shirts with the group's logo or life-affirming messages such as "#endoverdose" and "We Do Recover."

Monthly meetings on the first Thursday of each month from 6:30-8 p.m. are open to anyone. Most of the people who show up to talk about the group's work are family of people who use drugs, but a gathering also might find a man (or woman) in recovery sitting next to a woman (or man) who works in the field of substance abuse.

Active users are welcomed to meetings on the last Thursday each month from 6-9 p.m. These meetings are closed to the public. Participants have snacks (and sometimes a meal), fun, and a little education. Free Hepatitis C testing is available on the last Thursday of each month.

A typical supply bag for syringe exchange participants includes:
◊   40 syringes
◊   3 tourniquets

- ◊ Sterile water
- ◊ 5 sterile, disposable cookers
- ◊ 40 alcohol wipes
- ◊ 40-50 cotton pellets
- ◊ 5 or 6 condoms
- ◊ A sharps container
- ◊ Narcan, if needed
- ◊ Participants with infections also receive wipes, bandages, and Epsom salts.

Contact: Kelly Link, 336-465-1431 or kellyalink@outlook. com; Ashley Hedrick, 336-633-8974 or sincerelyashley85@ yahoo.com. Donations can be made via Paypal.me/ CommUNITYHopeAllianc (no "e").

LIVES
LOST
TOO SOON

'Breathtakingly beautiful'

Claudia Marini keeps her daughter's memory alive via Maddie's Mission

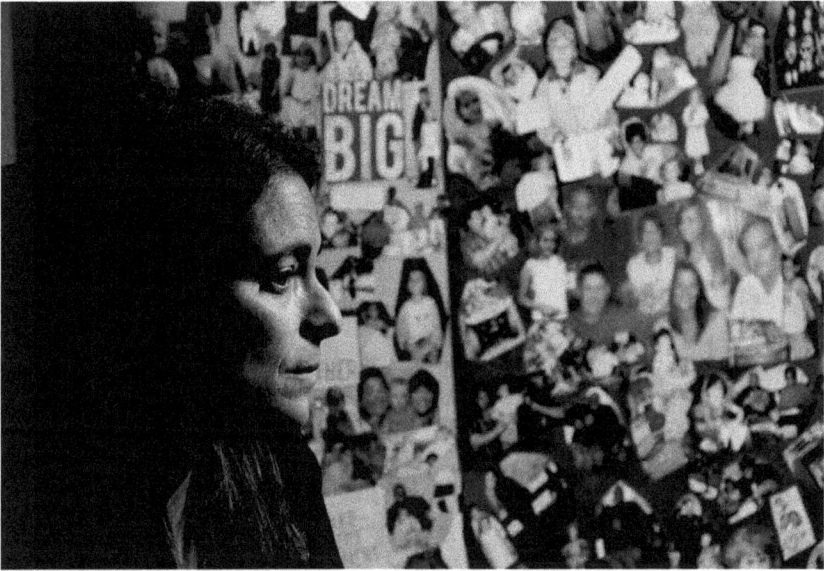

TELL THEM THEY ARE LOVED – Claudia Marini tells parents to let children who are struggling know they are loved. 'Don't forget, even when they're at their worst, or they're being horrible, or yelling, or screaming, to constantly just tell them you love them, and to give them that extra hug.' (Photograph by Paul Church/Courtesy The Courier-Tribune)

Four days after Christmas in 2016, a call to Claudia Marini's home east of Asheboro shattered the holiday cheer: Her daughter, Maddie, had overdosed.

Marini knew what to do. She shifted into got-to-go gear, never mind that she was laid up, recuperating from hip surgery a week earlier.

"We had gotten the phone call so often," Marini says, "I knew the routine, sadly, which is no routine any parent, anyone, should have to go through."

The things she needed to do: Get dressed; put up the dogs; get in the car; drive as fast as you can to the hospital; and then have the conversation, the same conversation as every other time: I love you, Maddie. This has got to stop.

21

But this time the caller said: "Don't come. We're working on her."

Waiting for the second call was excruciating. When it came, Marini remembers the look on her best friend's face as he walked into the room where she sat on the edge of the couch, her hands clasply tightly together, tense: "Let's go," she said. "We need to go."

She remembers Ken shaking his head and then the words, "She's gone. She didn't make it." Everything after that is a blur. "It's a really good thing that I went into shock," she says, "because I really have no doubt: I would have died when I heard that news. I would have died. I wanted to die."

There are still days when she goes through the motions from sunup to sundown. Sometimes in the stillness of the night, she cannot believe Maddie is gone.

"There's this unbelievable desperation of wanting her back so bad – and actually trying to figure out how to make that happen, and then, coming full circle, and realizing and telling myself that it can't happen. I don't even have the words to explain the hell that it feels like internally. And the pain."

Madison Bailey Marini died December 29, 2016, in the bathroom of the fast-food restaurant where she worked in the Stokes County town of King. Paramedics arrived too late.

She was 22.

Captivating and beautiful

After Maddie's death, Marini talked to newspaper and television reporters because she wanted news stories to be more than matter-of-fact accounts that another young person had died of an overdose.

She wanted the world to know who her daughter was. That her addiction did not define her. That she had a captivating personality and loved to sing. That she was someone's child. That she was loved. That she had dreams of becoming a forensic anthropologist. That her grandmother lovingly called her "Bones" because she spent so much time watching the TV show – about a forensic anthropologist – by that name.

"When Maddie walked into a room, just something happened," Marini says. "She just commanded that room. She was breathtakingly beautiful."

The people in a room might not remember her name later, or even know it, Marini says, but they would remember Maddie.

To keep her daughter's memory alive – and to raise money

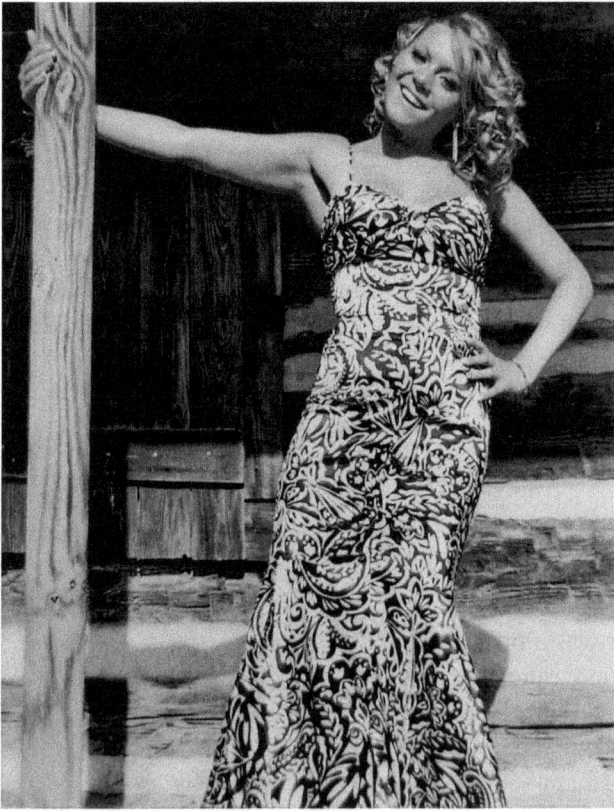

FULL OF LIFE – Madison Bailey Marini was 22 when she died of an overdose in 2016. 'When Maddie walked into a room, just something happened,' her mother says. 'She just commanded that room. She was breathtakingly beautiful.' (Contributed photo)

and awareness in the fight against substance abuse – Marini established Maddie's Mission and Maddie's Miles 5K, both of which help fund a Winston-Salem nonprofit called Phoenix Rising Inc. Its mission is to support drug court in Forsyth County; to fund treatment; and to launch awareness campaigns. Marini sits on the Phoenix Rising board of directors.

Treatment was not an option given to Maddie the last time she was in court. On that court date in October 2016, a few days before her 22nd birthday, Marini says her daughter was "fed up with being sick and tired" and ready to go to rehab.

Marini asked to talk to the judge. She wanted to tell him a little about Maddie and her desire to get help. Maddie's attorney presented the request. The judge brushed it off, saying that a defendant older than 18 did not need her mother speaking for her. As for treatment, he added, when he sent Maddie to jail, she

23

would get clean.

The jail was overcrowded, and Maddie was released early on her promise to get a job and show up every week for a drug test. She got a job at Taco Bell in the town where she was living with her grandparents.

In the few weeks she was there, she received an award from a district manager for being an exemplary employee. She seemed to be doing well. The old Maddie was back.

And then she was gone. Marini believes that if the judge had made a different decision in October, a decision to mandate rehab, it might have saved Maddie's life in December.

ADHD, drugs

Young Maddie tried ballet but was too fidgety to hold delicate poses. Soccer was more her liking, running up and down a field under the open sky.

But singing was her biggest thing, a talent she displayed in a youth community chorale and the school chorus. She enjoyed posting singing videos on Faccbook and counting the "likes" despite

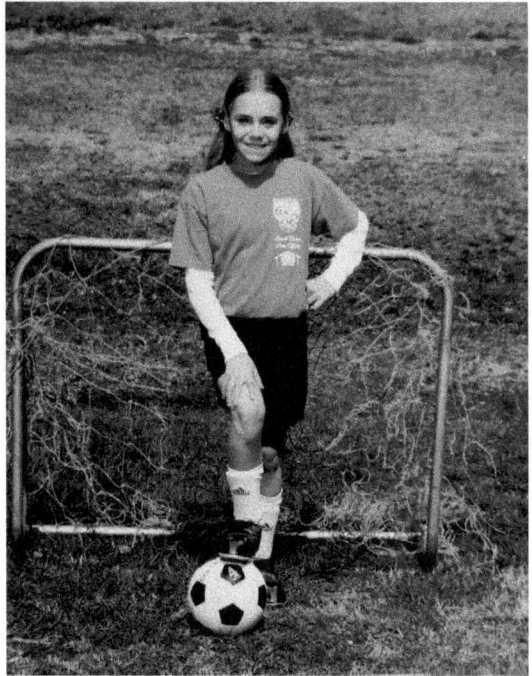

FULL OF ENERGY – Maddie Marini loved to play soccer but singing was her favorite thing to do. (Contributed photo)

her mother's lectures that something shared on the Internet is forever. Today, Marini is grateful for those videos.

Schoolwork came easy to Maddie, but she was tagged as a problem in the first grade. She was too loud. She did not like naps. She could not sit quietly at her desk. Most every day, her teacher wrote notes about Maddie's transgressions. Maddie thought the teacher did not like her. Soon she did not like going to school.

Maddie was diagnosed with ADHD, attention deficit

hyperactivity disorder.

"As a mom," Marini says, "when she was in school and having difficulty, we took her to the doctor, and they put her on medication."

Maddie and her mom went to therapy together, and Maddie had individual sessions, which she continued off and on into her high school years.

Marini regrets the decision to put Maddie on medication.

"She was just unique in a great way. Unfortunately, we don't really foster that in kids. We want them to be a certain way."

"… But you don't know what you don't know 'til sometimes it's too late. I thought I was doing what was best for Maddie. I didn't want her to get in trouble anymore. I didn't want her to feel that way when she went to school."

Marini wonders if the drugs Maddie took as a child, and well into her teens, contributed to future struggles with substance abuse.

"What a lot of people don't realize is that Ritalin and all that medication is very much addictive," she says. "And doctors don't do a good job of helping kids and adults wean off of that and find other alternatives."

Starting to spiral

Depression and anxiety dogged Maddie in middle school.

Once again, she did not want to go to school. She did not feel like she fit in. She often lashed out at her family. Again, Marini turned to professionals. "We did hospitalize her because we didn't know what else to do. It was one of the hardest things I ever had to do."

When Maddie was discharged, she was carrying a paper bag filled with medications. Then, Marini thought she was doing all the right things to help; now, she wonders. "It was just this circle, this vicious circle, that she could never get out of."

Maddie lost interest in soccer around the same time her mom caught her smoking cigarettes. Marini was shocked. Maddie, the athlete, would never do something to impair her ability to sprint the length of the field for hours. Maddie skipped practices, so, on game day, the coach kept her on the bench. She quit.

Marini decided that a small private school might serve Maddie better than public school and enrolled her in a Catholic school in Winston-Salem. Maddie loved the idea because she would get to live with her grandparents in King.

And, she did better, until high school, when she met a boy who was not a good influence. Marini had been missing Maddie, so they decided she would return home and go to Randolph Early College High School at Randolph Community College.

As she got older, Maddie sometimes stopped taking her ADHD medication for stretches of time. By high school, she stopped altogether.

"She never liked taking the medications," Marini says. "She didn't feel like it made a difference." Looking back, Marini says she's not sure the drugs had much of an affect either, besides making her daughter sleepy. Of course, when Maddie was sleepy, she was quiet in school, the desired effect.

Also, in high school, Maddie started self-medicating, but her mother did not know that yet. The boy Marini thought they had left behind in Stokes County started showing up in Asheboro. Sometimes, when Marini thought Maddie was in school, she was spending the day with him. One Thanksgiving, Maddie ran away; she went to the boy's house.

Maddie's moods fluctuated. Sometimes she was sad and unhappy, sometimes volatile and angry. Marini attributed the occasional sadness and anger to teenage hormones and the social trauma of high school.

Then Maddie stopped worrying about how she looked. She slept more. She picked at her fingers, but that was not too alarming; it was a habit she'd also had as a child. She brushed aside questions about sores her mom noticed on her body. It was just acne, Maddie said.

Before long she was struggling with her studies. At a parent/ teacher conference her sophomore year, a teacher noted that Maddie was starting to spiral. Had Marini considered that Maddie might be using drugs? She knew Maddie was smoking, Marini said, assuring the teacher that they were working on that.

The teacher said Maddie was exhibiting classic signs of someone using methamphetamine. Marini was blindsided.

"It felt like I had been knocked down by a bulldozer."

'They had a pain'

Maddie denied it, but the teacher was right.

"This was just a whole world I knew nothing about," Marini says, "so I didn't know the signs."

In trying to fit in, to find her niche, Marini says, Maddie gravitated to the wrong crowd, kids with similar issues, kids who were struggling, kids who made bad choices.

Years later, when Maddie was deep into addiction, Marini

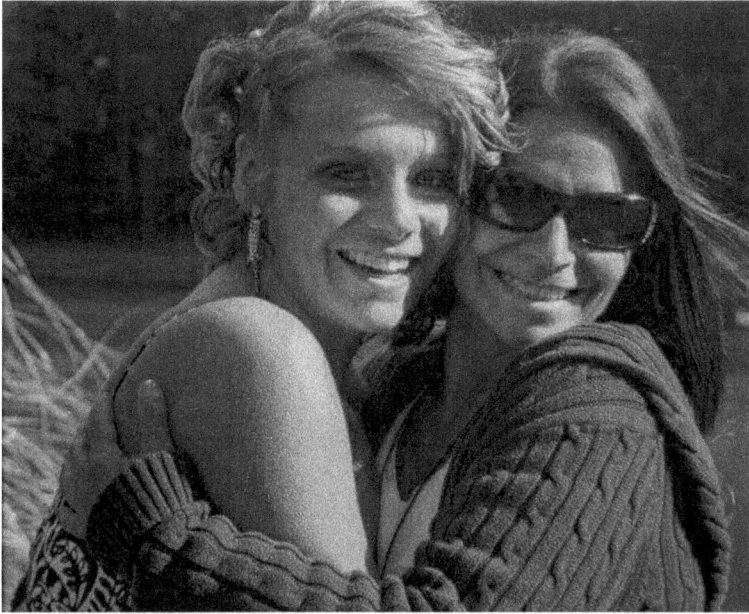

MOM AND DAUGHTER – Maddie and Claudia Marini share a joyous hug. Maddie had dreams of becoming a forensic anthropologist. Her grandmother called her 'Bones' because Maddie spent so much time watching the TV show by that name. (Contributed photo)

talked to her about her choice of friends. Maddie replied that her friends were the only people who understood her.

Marini was frustrated. "I thought, gosh, how could those be the only people that understand you? Those aren't people making good choices."

She gets it now. "They had a commonality. They had a pain. They shared it. They understood. And there just wasn't enough resources and understanding at the time to pull those kids out of where they were."

Maddie's drug use progressed to pain pills, eventually to heroin. She went to jail for petty crimes and probation violation. She stole things from her mom and grandparents she could pawn for money or trade for drugs. She was caught shoplifting.

Marini and her family tried smothering love, nurturing her daughter in every way they knew how, and tough love, kicking Maddie out for not following the rules. Nothing worked.

Maddie knew she could come home, but she also knew her mother was not going to allow her to use drugs, so she bounced from place to place, staying with her grandparents, or with friends.

Marini knows of four times her daughter overdosed. Once she

27

was stabilized at the hospital after an overdose, Maddie would be given a list of treatment facilities and released.

"We'd always say, 'If you let her go, by the time we make the phone calls, by the time we find a bed, she's gonna be sick.' And that's what happened every time. Every single time."

Drug users call it dopesick: Maddie would go into withdrawal – her body craving whatever drug currently had her in its grip.

She was in and out of treatment. In a span of four years, she checked into one facility four or five times and was kicked out of another for not following rules. Whenever she had been in treatment for a while, the "old" Maddie would resurface, happy and smiling.

"When they're using for so long," Marini says, "they become this other person that's not the person that you raised and remember. It's just this other person. And when they get clean, the person you remember comes back."

'My time to shine'

Christmas Day 2016 is the last time Marini saw Maddie alive.

She was the old Maddie, not the sullen and argumentative Maddie, but the Maddie whose smile lit up rooms. She complained about gaining weight, a good sign. A "skinny" Maddie usually meant she was using drugs.

On this day, Maddie was plump and laughing as she opened presents. She rushed from the room to try on every new piece of clothing and gleefully returned to show her family.

"It was like she was 5 years old," Marini says. "We hadn't seen Maddie like that in a long time."

Twenty days earlier, on December 5, Maddie wrote her last journal entry – ninety-eight words full of the optimism and hope her family saw on Christmas Day:

This journal is going to be all about my new independent life and my time line of me achieving everything I set my heart on. This is the first time I have been truly single and doing everything on my own.

As of right now I am still on probation, have a pending charge, no license or car, not in school and still living at home. I work at Taco Bell. My goal is by the end of this journal all of that will change. I am done being a screw up. It is my time to shine.

'Tell them you love them'

Marini says she hopes that, through Maddie's Mission, she can offer a voice that changes a parent's life or the life of someone struggling with addiction.

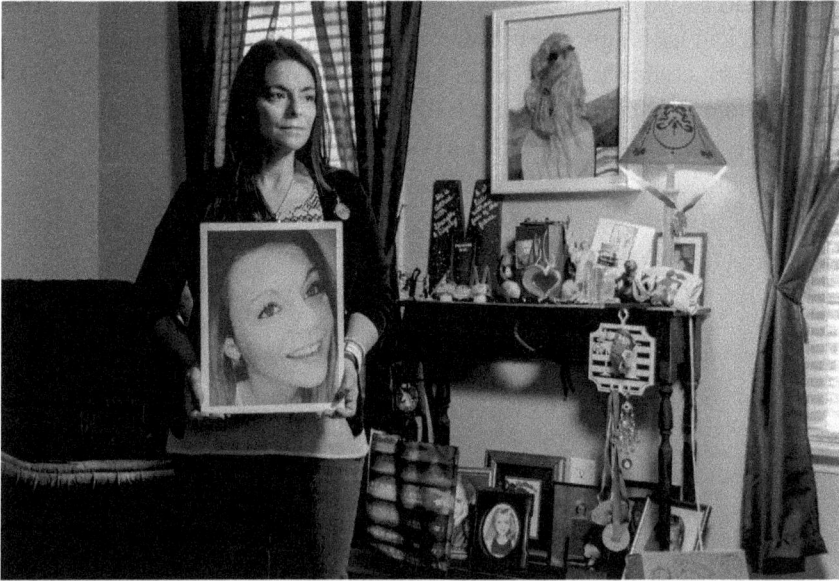

FOR MADDIE – A table in Claudia Marini's home east of Asheboro holds photographs and things that remind her of her daughter, Maddie, who died in 2016. A framed portrait on the wall features a lock of Maddie's long, blonde hair. (Photo by Paul Church/Courtesy The Courier-Tribune)

She encourages parents to ask questions and to have uncomfortable conversations with their children if something does not seem right. It's better to make them angry, she says, than to regret doing nothing.

But, above all, let children who are struggling know they are loved.

"Don't forget, even when they're at their worst," she says, "or they're being horrible, or yelling, or screaming, to constantly just tell them you love them, and to give them that extra hug."

In the early days of Maddie's struggles, Marini thought she knew the answer to the question of whether addiction is a choice or a disease. She thought Maddie simply needed to make better decisions. Now she says she understands that Maddie, and others shackled by drugs, suffer from sickness, mental and physical, that requires professional help.

"It's just so damn difficult," Marini says. "It is so difficult. And sometimes it is just easier to stay in the throes of it and live that life than to go through the hoops of what it takes to get clean."

In the perfect world, she envisions fully funded treatment, no questions asked, for those who want it, start-to-finish programs that encompass detox, rehab, counseling, and life skills to help participants get back on their feet.

Maddie wanted to quit.

"It had nothing to do with her not wanting to," Marini says, "but she couldn't, and it wasn't because she didn't try. Nobody would ever willingly choose to live the kind of life somebody who's on drugs and addicted lives. It's horrible. It's absolutely horrible."

Mom on a mission
Susan Hunt intends for her son's death to make a difference

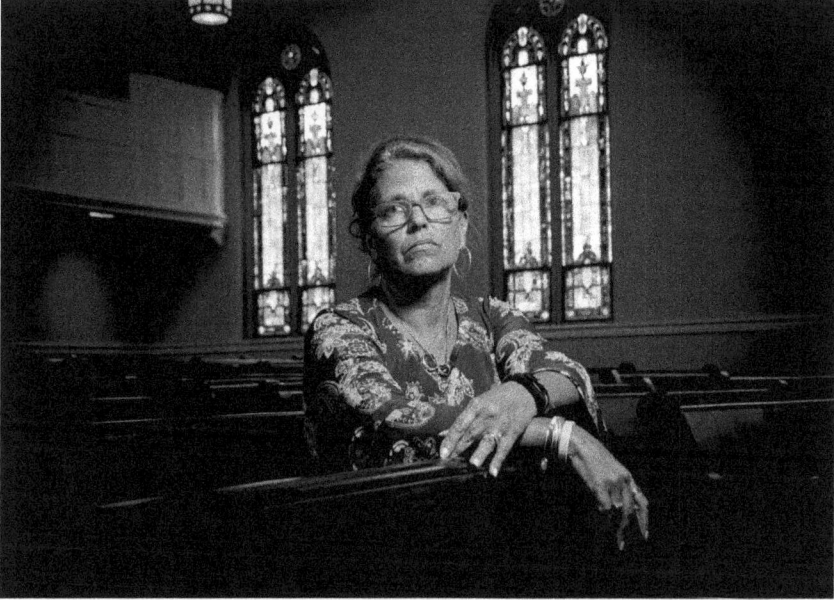

POWERHOUSE ADVOCATE – Susan Hunt plans to spread the word about the dangers of drug addiction to young people, parents, and the world. Her son, Keaton Scott Hunt, died June 12, 2019, after an overdose. (Photograph by Paul Church/Courtesy The Courier-Tribune)

The last communication Susan Hunt had with her son was a text message on Monday, June 10, a quarter of an hour before he overdosed.

Just two weeks earlier, Keaton had been kicked out of an inpatient drug treatment program for breaking rules.

Keaton had cut the grass that Monday afternoon, and Susan texted to say that it looked good. She asked what he was doing. Riding around with his girlfriend, he replied and sent a picture.

She reminded him that he had had a court date the next morning. She also reminded him that if his probation officer happened to be in court, she could ask him to take a drug test.

"You know that, right?" she said.

"Yes, lol," he replied.

Security camera video shows Keaton walking into the bathroom of an Asheboro fast-food restaurant about 15 minutes later. About 20 minutes after that, a city police officer called Susan to tell her that Keaton had overdosed in the bathroom.

Emergency rescue personnel worked on Keaton for some time before they detected a heartbeat. After a scan at Randolph Health showed no brain activity, he was transferred to Novant Health Forsyth Medical Center in Winston-Salem for organ procurement

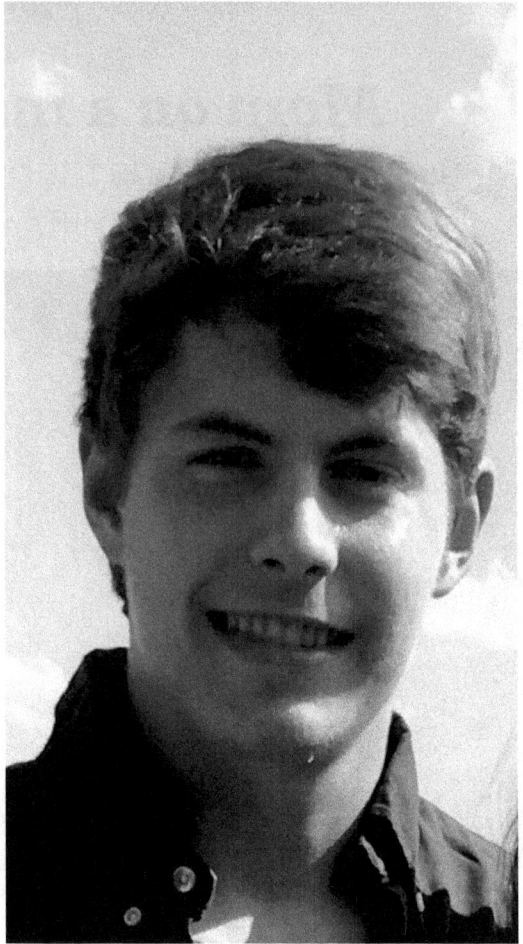

Keaton Scott Hunt 1999-2019

arranged with the help of Carolina Donor Services.

Keaton's heart was transplanted to a man in his 60s who has an adult son. The man works in sales.

A woman in her 50s received Keaton's liver and left kidney. She's married and works in project management and enjoys dog rescue work, crafts, and gardening. Her message to Keaton's family: "The gratitude I feel is overwhelming. I will do the very best I can to honor and protect your loved one's memory."

His pancreas and right kidney went to a man in his 30s. He enjoys music, computers, and gaming. His message: "Thank you. Thank you so much."

His lungs were recovered for research.

The last time she saw her son, medical personnel were wheeling him to an operating room to recover his organs.

"I told Keaton when he got on the elevator, next time I put my hand on your heart it's going to be in somebody else."

She cried in a recent interview as she shared the good news about the successful transplants. She has cried every day since drugs killed Keaton Scott Hunt, her only son. He was 20 years old.

'With the wrong kids'

A younger Keaton played sports. He was a pitcher in baseball and a quarterback in football. He announced, at 12 or 13, that he wanted to stop playing because he did not want to get hurt.

"I really attribute this whole drug journey he went on to him stopping sports," Susan said in a recent interview. "When he stopped playing sports, he stopped having that core group of friends to hang around with … he just started hanging around with the wrong kids."

Born under the sign of Aquarius, Keaton loved water. His mama threw him off the diving board at the YMCA when he was 9 months old and told him to swim. Susan pointed out that she was a water baby instructor, so Keaton already knew how to swim, and there was someone in the water to help him if he needed it.

But he did not need help. He swam.

He was a PADI-certified scuba diver by 10 and a Red Cross-certified lifeguard at 15. He was credited with making six saves as a lifeguard at the swimming pool at High Point City Lake park.

He attended First Youth at Asheboro's First United Methodist Church. The day before he overdosed, he was at Sunday service, like always unless he was working, and hugged the Rev. Lynda Ferguson. That was not unusual either. He had a giving heart, she said. Keaton shared his struggles with her: "He always told me the worst thing was what he was doing to his mom."

A people person, Keaton was especially popular with girls. In kindergarten, Keaton made a small poster for Cassie, a classmate with Down syndrome. He wrote on it that that Cassie was his best friend.

Last year, well over a decade removed from kindergarten, Cassie decided that she wanted Keaton to take her to homecoming at Uwharrie Charter Academy. When Keaton found out, he asked for a change in his work schedule to escort his longtime friend.

School did not much interest him, though he did well without

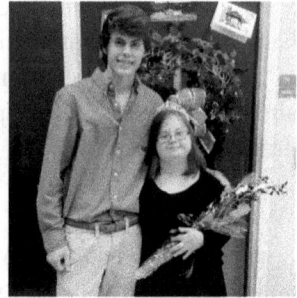

studying. His score on the ACT, a standardized test used for college admissions, placed him among the top 20 percent of test takers. He later told his mom that he was high when he took it.

Seeking higher highs

Keaton was 14 when he started smoking pot, but his parents did not know it then. They caught him when he was 15, but he deflected blame to another boy. A year later, they found marijuana in his truck and confronted him again. This time, Susan called a magistrate to report what they had found.

"What do you want me to do about it?" the magistrate asked her.

Now, Susan says she wishes she had called the police instead. If her son had been arrested, she said, it may have made a difference in his life.

Keaton's drug journey progressed to "dabbing" – heating and inhaling a waxy cannabis extract that's extremely high in THC, the psychoactive substance that produces the high. Many users employ handheld blow torches when dabbing. Keaton told his parents he used the torches found in his truck to start bonfires.

The litany of drugs he tried that Susan knows about included roxies (the street name for a prescription opioid painkiller) and synthetic weed. When she found what looked like black soot marks in a bathroom at her home, she thought it was residue from her daughter's mascara. Then she found black fingerprints on Keaton's bedroom door. He had been using black tar heroin.

After his death, Keaton's friends told her that Keaton had started using fentanyl to get high because the drugs he had been doing were not powerful enough. Fentanyl is a synthetic opioid that is 80-100 times stronger than morphine.

Dodging drug tests

Last year, Greensboro police found marijuana and a small bottle containing about four ounces of colored liquid in Keaton's truck. It was what's known as "liquid heroin," a concoction also known by street names such as lean and purple drank. It's a homemade mix of prescription-strength cough medicine, soft drinks, and fruit-flavored candy.

Among the charges Keaton faced – carrying as much as 27 years in prison – was one for trafficking in opiates because prescription cough syrup contains the opioid codeine. But he did not go to prison. Under a program for first offenders, he was placed on probation, required to have a drug assessment, and to comply with any recommendations.

Keaton later told his mother he started using heroin regularly because as a probationer he was subject to routine and random drug testing. Marijuana can be detected in the system much longer than heroin, weeks versus days.

Despite his efforts to beat the system, Keaton failed a drug test in April after smoking pot. He was arrested and spent six days in the Randolph County Jail, detoxing (from the heroin and whatever other drugs he had been using) on a mattress on the floor in a room in the booking area with four other men.

He was a candidate for admission to DART Cherry, a residential treatment facility in Goldsboro for probationers, Susan said, but that did not happen because he was released from custody due to a paperwork snafu.

"So," she said, "we started trying to find treatment centers."

Finding help

Susan, her sister, Keaton, and his girlfriend spent days calling treatment centers – 34 in all -- trying to find a place for him to go. There were no beds available. Susan found facilities in California that would take him, but his probation prohibited him from leaving the state. She also found a place in Greensboro that would take him if she paid $8,000 cash "just to get him in the door."

After he got out of jail, Susan had started doing drug tests at home. One day he failed the test, so, as she had told him she would do if he ever failed a drug test, she took him to a Greensboro hospital.

While they sat in the waiting room for the next six hours they cried together. He told her that all he ever wanted to do was smoke marijuana to calm his nerves, but after he started using heroin to dodge detection during drug tests, he could not stop.

"Keaton, this is going to be the beginning of you getting out of this," she told him.

But it wasn't. She thought hospital personnel would evaluate him, find out what drugs were in his system, and then get him to an appropriate place for treatment of his addiction. But during his exam Keaton said that he was not suicidal and did not need to detox. The hospital staff said all they could offer was a list of treatment facilities. Susan had already contacted most of them.

A friend finally located a small treatment center in Asheville that gave Keaton a spot. He went in early May. On the way, Keaton asked Susan to tell anyone who asked that he was working out of town. He did not want anyone to know the truth.

"They're going to think I'm a drug addict for the rest of my life," he said.

'Mama, come get me'

He seemed to have an epiphany of sorts after he had been in Asheville just a short time. "Mama, I can't believe how lucky I am because there are people in here who have lost everything," he told her. "I'll never take for granted the things you gave me."

But he did. After 25 days, Keaton called. "Mama," he said, "you have to come get me."

He was being kicked out of the treatment center because staff had found a bottle of urine in his room. Drug users sometimes substitute urine from people who do not use drugs to avoid positive drug tests.

Susan told Keaton she did not have to come get him – the family had already endured too much turmoil related to his drug use. She did not go to Asheville, but his girlfriend did.

Susan did not see him for three days after he was released, and then they talked for a long time. He wanted to come home. She asked if he had had drug cravings since leaving treatment. He told her he had not.

She thought that maybe what he had learned in three-plus weeks in Asheville would be enough to keep him on the right track if he found a job and worked an outpatient treatment program. He agreed to stay clean.

She did not find out until weeks after his death that he had overdosed in the days between his aborted rehab stay and his return home. She might never have known, but, since he was covered under her insurance, she got a bill from the hospital where he had spent nine hours.

She still does not know what happened then. Due to confidentiality laws, the hospital cannot tell her.

'Get them help'

Now she is on a mission. Several missions, in fact.

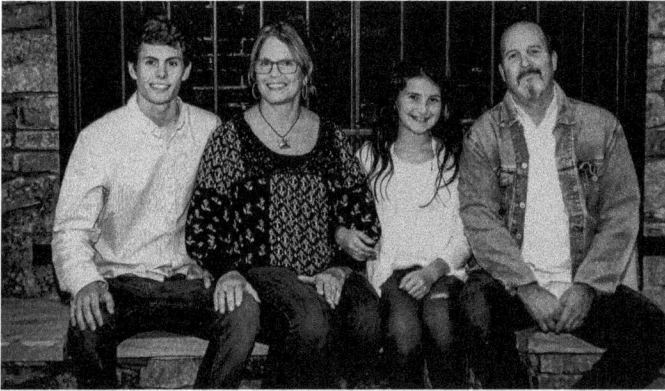

HAPPY OCCASION – Keaton Hunt, left, with his mother, Susan, his sister, Ella, and his father, Tim Campbell. (Contributed photo)

She wants young people to know they are playing Russian roulette if they use drugs, even marijuana because it may be laced with more deadly drugs.

"You can't do this stuff because it'll kill you. You try this one time, two times, it starts rewiring your brain, and you can't get away from this – and you're doing this to your family, and your parents and people that love you don't deserve this."

Susan wants parents to learn the signs of drug use.

"It's so hard to detect whether or not these kids are doing these drugs," she said. "If you start early, you can make a difference. When they're 18, it's so hard. "People have to stop the stigma. If your kids are using, you have to get them help."

And she wants Asheboro school officials to keep naloxone, a medication that blocks the effects of opioids, especially in overdose, at the high school – and to consider keeping it at the middle schools, too. Her message: "You guys better get your head out of the sand because somebody's going to die of an overdose."

She also plans to push for school programs that feature former drug users telling the ugly story of how drugs are killing people.

She's sure it could make a difference, as Keaton's death has.

Several young people have told her that Keaton's death opened their eyes to dangers they previously ignored:

"And then they all say, well, it's really made a difference now, 'cause if it can get Keaton, it can get any of us."

Addiction is like a dark cloud that comes in and consumes you, takes away your ability to make a choice and torments your soul.

'Sadness in my heart'

Anna Bigelow talks about addiction to save lives

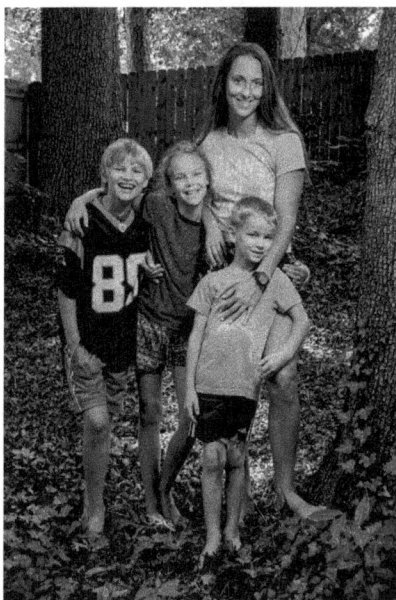

STILL STRONG – Anna Bigelow and her children, left to right, Bearik, Grace, and Maverick, pose for a family portrait at their home in Asheboro. Jason Bigelow, husband and father, died of an overdose in May of 2018. (Photograph by Paul Church/Courtesy The Courier-Tribune)

This story by Annette Jordan appeared in The (Asheboro, N.C.) Courier-Tribune in May 2018. It is reprinted with permission.

The opioid crisis. You've heard those words a lot lately. According to a CDC Morbidity and Mortality Report released this March, drug overdose deaths claimed 63,632 Americans in 2016, nearly two-thirds involving opioids. Closer to home, in just the first four months of 2018 alone, 157 suspected overdoses and 19 deaths have been reported in Randolph County. Fatalities have ranged from an 18-year-old male to a 65-year-old male.

Those are the numbers.

Here's one of the faces.

On May 1, Jason Bigelow's body was discovered in an abandoned house near High Point. He had been missing from his Asheboro home for a week, and while the autopsy results are still pending, his wife, Anna, has no doubt what the cause of death was.

On April 30, the day before he was found, she posted this on Facebook in one angry, anguished burst:

"My husband is missing and no one has heard from him in 6 days. Even in his darkest of times he would have not gone that long without communication. It's hard to know what to feel, stricken with fear, paralyzed with worry.

"Addiction, it's the one word no one wants to talk about, like a dark secret, but it's destroyed so many lives. To be honest I'm not mad at Jason. If anything I'm mad at the community who looked at him so differently because of his addictions and faults. I feel like God's grace has never run out on him, but our grace ran out for him. People think here we go again, or it's another relapse, or if he loved his family then why couldn't he just quit. I will say this, I have never once doubted Jason's love for me or the kids.

"Addiction is like a dark cloud that comes in and consumes you, takes away your ability to make a choice and torments your soul. I apologize for my brutal honesty, but maybe that's what this town needs, not small talks, pretend smiles and bull****. But truth, our struggles, our weaknesses."

***

Anna Bigelow doesn't have all the answers. She doesn't know if anything could have saved Jason, but she believes some of the ways to put a dent in the opioid epidemic is to talk honestly about addiction. Locally, it would help to have more transitional programs for addicts, she believes, and if people could gravitate to more natural remedies, diet and exercise, instead of medication, maybe that could make a difference, too.

She hopes that sharing her very painful personal story might help someone struggling now.

***

Jason and Anna's story begins at Appalachian State University where they were students. One day in the library, he walked up to the pretty co-ed, teasing her that she needed to leave because she was "distracting him and he wasn't getting any work done."

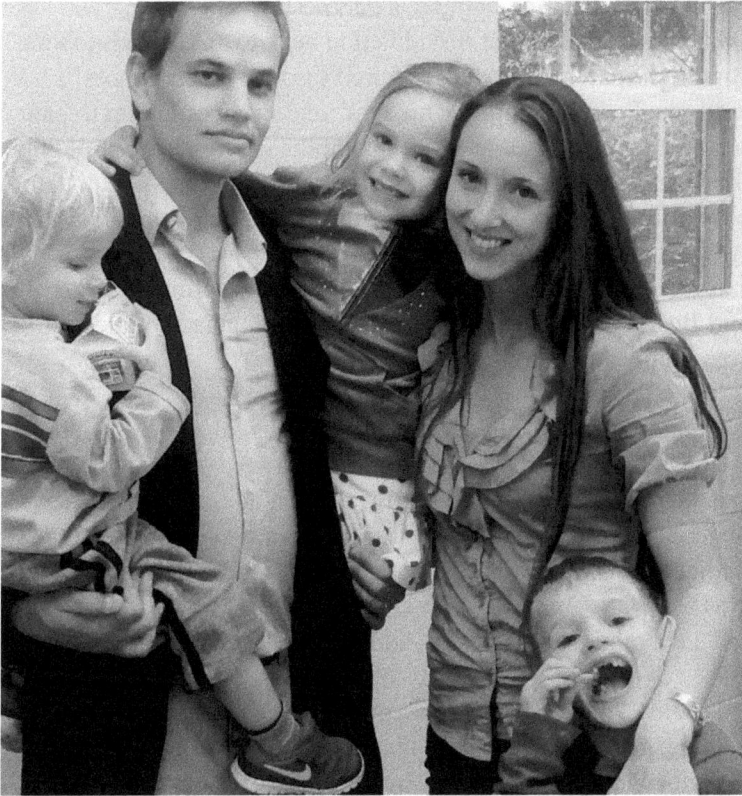

FAMILY PORTRAIT – Jason and Anna Bigelow and their children, left to right, Maverick, Grace, and Bearik smile for the camera. (Contributed photo)

From there, Jason pursued her romantically, and while she was at first reluctant, soon found herself falling in love.

"He'd take me to waterfalls, take me hiking, take me to sunsets. He always took me to beautiful places," she says.

On Jan. 14, 2007, they married in one of those beautiful places, "a big cliff that overlooks all of Boone," the very place he had asked her to be his girlfriend.

The couple shared a love of the outdoors, which they would impart to their children, Bearik, Grace and Maverick. Hiking, riding mountain bikes, snowboarding, jumping off waterfalls, hanging hammocks over cliffs — those were good times. Anna loved the way Jason was easy-going and non-judgmental, "the most loving, accepting person you could meet." He had a heart of gold, family would later write in his obituary in The Courier-Tribune, an unforgettable smile and an energy that brought light to any dark room.

***

But underneath the light lay a darkness.

She traces the seed of his addiction back to an early childhood condition (paresthesia) that required Jason to "wear braces, kind like Forrest Gump, on his legs" and introduced him to pain medication. The disease didn't take full root, however, until after they married and he underwent a hip replacement — and lots of pain pills — followed by severe, life-threatening complications. And even more pain-killers.

By the time they moved to Asheboro in the spring of 2007 and Bearik's birth in June, Jason's medicating had spiraled into something dangerous.

So had Anna's.

"I started using with him," she says, drugs like Oxycodone, cocaine, whatever they could find. "We started shooting up together. Now that I look back I wasn't an addict. I was an abuser. I was trying to deal with being in a relationship with an addict and the only way I could connect with him or be with him was use with him."

They both lost their jobs ... and worse.

***

On July 9, 2008, Jason robbed the High Country Bank in Foscoe, a small town near Boone, of $15,000. Armed with a toy BB gun and wearing a mask, he went into the bank while Anna stayed outside with their son. She then drove "the getaway car" to the beach, but the couple soon learned there were warrants out for their arrest. A witness had seen the two in the bank before the robbery and recognized the dress Anna was wearing.

On the advice of an attorney and after handing Bearik over to Tina Goss, Jason's mom back in Asheboro, the couple turned themselves in.

"They stripped us down, hosed us off, threw us into padded cells. They thought we were suicidal," Anna says. "We had a miraculous encounter with Christ on the same day," a moment that gave her the strength for what was to follow, she says: Pleading guilty when she was 7 months pregnant with their daughter; delivering Grace in prison; serving 2 1/2 years in a Tallahassee, Fla., prison while Jason served his time in a N.J. correctional facility; and being released on Jan. 14, 2011 (their fourth anniversary).

At 25, while still in prison, Jason underwent yet another hip replacement.

"It was dislocated in prison. His hip (replacement) was also recalled. It was releasing toxic metals and causing complications in people who received it."

Right before Christmas 2011, he reunited with the family. They moved into a rented house in Asheboro and Jason took work he could find as a delivery boy.

***

For awhile, life was good. Jason remained sober for five years, launched a marketing company, enjoyed a fit lifestyle (he was a weight lifting enthusiast) — and then Anna began to notice the telltale signs of addiction. He began, as she put it, "to invite things back into his life."

To rehab he went; then a halfway house; and the cycle continued ... more overdosing, more bouts of guilt and shame over relapsing; more health problems and surgeries; more painkillers; and inevitably, the loss of his business. Humiliated, the man Anna described as a "marketing genius" was forced to take odd jobs, construction, driving a lumber truck.

"It was like he could never get out of it. I was starting to understand more. I was starting to see this wasn't as simple as: 'Why can't you just quit?' or 'You don't love me enough.' ... I started focusing on myself. I began to realize his addiction had nothing to do with me and my happiness had nothing to do with him. I had to find my own path."

She hopes that path will one day lead to becoming a physical therapist. This summer, Anna, who works as a physical therapy aide at Deep River Rehabilitation and is a personal trainer at her own business, plans to apply to the physical therapy program at Guilford Technical Community College.

Her career choice, she says, was inspired by watching Jason's courage in learning to walk again.

***

Jason went missing on Tuesday, April 24. Earlier that day, there had been a fight over his drug use with Anna and an ominous plea to his mom and sister, Jamie Bigelow: "Just let me go!"

Initially, no one was alarmed, the family being all too familiar with his habit of disappearing for a day or two.

But on Wednesday night, Anna had a strange experience. Suddenly jarred away by the sound of her husband's voice, she heard, "Anna, Anna, come on!," so clearly, she actually got out of bed and looked out the window thinking Jason was trying to get into the house. No one was there.

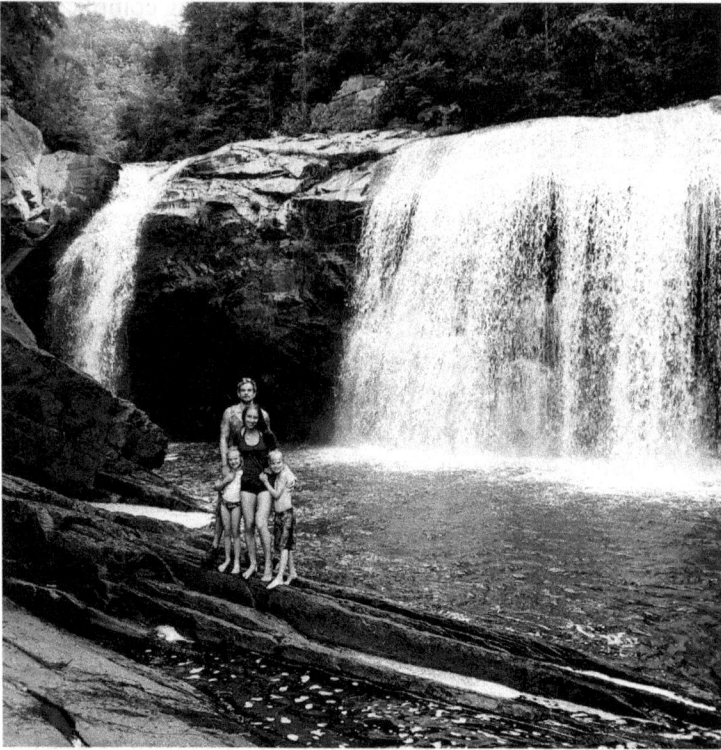

OUTDOOR LOVE – Jason and Anna Bigelow and their children Grace and Bearik stop for a picture with a waterfall roaring in the background. (Contributed photo)

She began to pray for his safety, as a premonition "deep in my heart" began to grow that something was terribly wrong, that this time the well-worn pattern of disappearing for a day or two might be something more serious. On May 1, his body was found at the abandoned house, propped up against the screened-in porch, overlooking a pond. The 35-year-old had been dead several days.

Anna believes he died the night she heard his voice.

***

"Words cannot even begin to express the pain, the sadness in my heart," she wrote on Facebook the next day.

"This seems so unreal, I never thought I would lose someone I love so much so young. I can't imagine growing old without him going through life with the kids without him. Yesterday morning my daily bible verse said, 'But you are a chosen race, a royal priesthood, a holy nation, a people for his own possession, that you may proclaim the excellencies of him who called you out of darkness into his marvelous light.' 1 Peter 2:9

"No matter how much it hurts I know Jason was telling me he had been called out of his darkness and into God's Marvelous light.

"I imagine this will hurt my whole life and it brings me some hope and peace to think that one day when I go to heaven, Jason will be there holding my hand. I know this life is but brief in comparison to eternity. God give me the strength to get through and to let my candle not grow dim with sorrow but brighter through the darkness and pain."

* * *

What Anna says ...

It has been one year and four months since my husband passed.

I still have dreams where I relive those events all over again, trying to find Jason, never making it to him fast enough, always too late. Then I awaken to grief-stricken, cannot-breathe, I-have-lost-the-love-of-my-life moments.

On those mornings, I want to hide under my sheets and never awaken to the day without him. When Jason passed, a part of me wanted to hide under my sheets forever, to run as far away from addiction as possible.

If you have been a part of it, whether loving someone or struggling with it yourself, you know this feeling. Addiction can be absolutely terrifying.

Finding your loved one passed out on the floor with a bag of needles; not knowing when, or if, someone will come home; being in constant fear of life and death; being let down time and time again.

It's miserable.

So that's what we do. We run from it. We don't talk about it. And, if we do, it's always in some negative light:

"Did you hear about so and so, I thought they were doing so good."

"Yep, that's addiction."

I am not saying it doesn't hurt. You have seen addiction take and destroy life, so, yes, running from it, never mentioning it, seems completely reasonable. But I decided I am not hiding

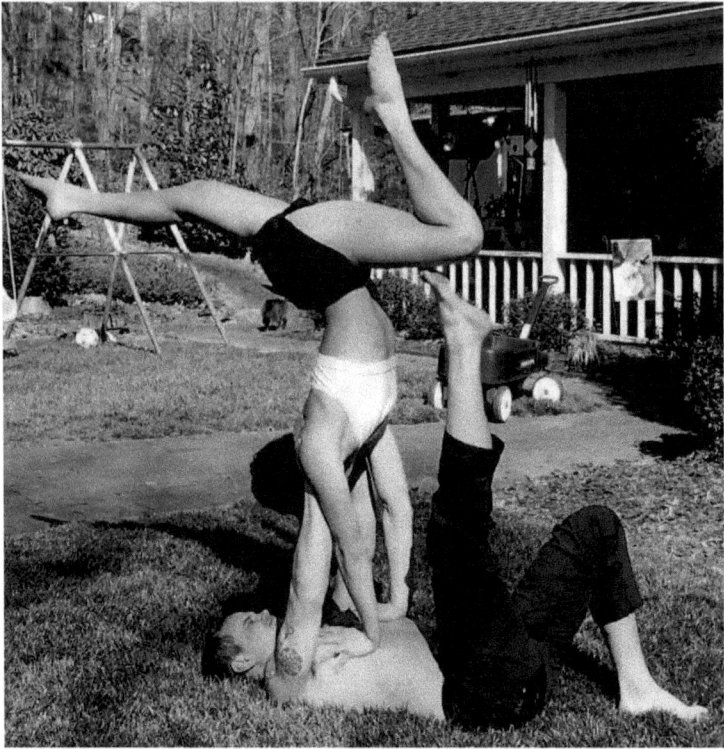

IN SHAPE – Anna and Jason Bigelow shared a love of physical fitness and the outdoors, including hiking, snowboarding, riding mountain bikes, and more. (Contributed photo)

under my sheets anymore. I am not hiding behind my fears, shame, guilt, could haves or what ifs. I am here to take a stand, to give the face of addiction a new name, to bring light into darkness.

So, what do I do? I talk about it, but I don't talk about it like it's some horrible story I am a victim in. I shift my perspective. I stop looking at the disease and look at the person. I stop being the victim and become the victor.

You will never hear me say the day Jason died was the worst day of my life. Maybe it was the most difficult, but you will never hear me say the day he decided to use was the biggest mistake of his life because – even through the pain, the guilt, the shame, the heartache – there is something absolutely beautiful.

I experienced more life with Jason than ever before. I loved like never before. And I am who I am because of it.

So yes, even through it all, I am thankful. Every second of every day I am thankful for you, Jason Bigelow. My life is lived with passion and love because of the way you loved me.

I will scream from the mountaintops, from valleys, from oceans and streams.

I will let the world know that people are not defined by their addiction, their loss, or their shame.

They are beautiful.

They are loved.

And they are here for a purpose.

BREAKING
FREE

A new Tonya was born in the mountains. The old one really died. I'm not the same person as I used to be.

'It's agonizing'

Twins in addiction: Tonya Waugh misses her sister, Toni Smith

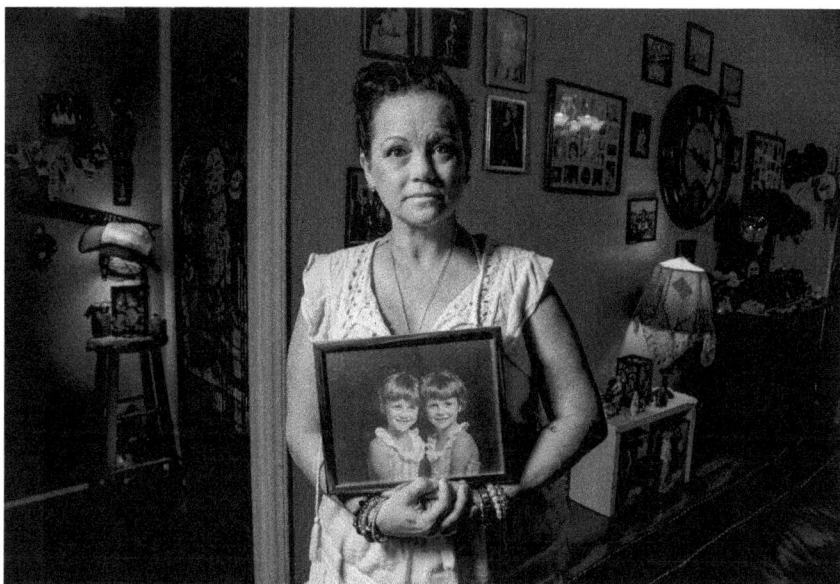

PAINFUL SEPARATION – Tonya Waugh holds a photograph of herself and her identical twin, Toni Smith, when they were young. Each twin battled addiction. Toni died from an overdose on April 4, 2015. (Photograph by Paul Church/Courtesy The Courier-Tribune)

Tonya and Toni Shinn entered the world six minutes apart on the day after Christmas in 1972. The pair shared the sort of bond felt only, perhaps, by twins.

"If you messed with one of us – even if we were fighting a behind-the-scenes type thing – you always got the other sister – it was bad," Tonya Waugh, the older sibling, says today. "We looked out for each other."

After they grew up and married – Toni at 19 and Tonya a year later – the sisters lived just a couple of miles from each other. The identical twins and their husbands got together often; the sisters talked on the phone every morning.

The conversations ended when Toni Smith died from an overdose on April 4, 2015. She was 42.

"I can feel a separation from her now," Tonya says. "It's agonizing, really."

Tonya says she does not know the details of her sister's struggle with drugs. It's not the kind of thing sisters, even twins, typically discuss with each other – or with anyone else. Drug users hide their addictions. Or try to. Or think they are hiding them.

It's what Tonya did for years when she was drinking and taking too many prescription pills. But she has been clean since she overdosed and went to rehab in the summer of 2013.

She tried to save her sister, too.

"I couldn't save her, no matter how hard I tried. You cannot save anybody. They have to want it for themselves. And as much as I would have laid down my life for her, she had to do it on her own."

Which Shinn Twin?

The girls were 6 when their father, Tony, died of a cocaine overdose at the age of 24. With their mother deemed incompetent, they lived with their paternal grandparents for a time before an aunt and uncle took custody and raised them on a horse farm in the northeastern corner of Randolph County.

Waugh says their home life was not an easy one. "My worst nightmare" is how she describes her upbringing: "I wasn't ever told I was loved growing up."

Most people could not tell the girls apart. A common question they heard was "which Shinn Twin are you?" Sometimes they fooled teachers, and once a boyfriend, by switching clothes and swapping places (as soon as they were old enough to make their own choices, they never dressed alike).

In high school, they both drank a little and smoked marijuana occasionally, but each had her own circle of friends and other interests that kept them busy.

Tonya tended toward gymnastics and cheerleading (she was chief cheerleader for two years in high school); Toni showed horses and sang in school chorus. Their senior year, both were on the cheerleading squad, and both sang.

A functioning addict

Tonya was diagnosed with Crohn's disease when she was 16 and with fibromyalgia when she was 26. Crohn's is an inflammatory bowel disease; fibromyalgia is a chronic rheumatic condition that causes pain throughout the body.

She says she did not start overusing medications prescribed to alleviate pain, including morphine and an opiate painkiller named Vicodin, until after her daughter was born in 1998. The stresses of motherhood amplified the symptoms of her health conditions, and she needed even more relief from pain.

When Tonya suspected she might have a problem, she decided to stop taking them. She felt awful but did

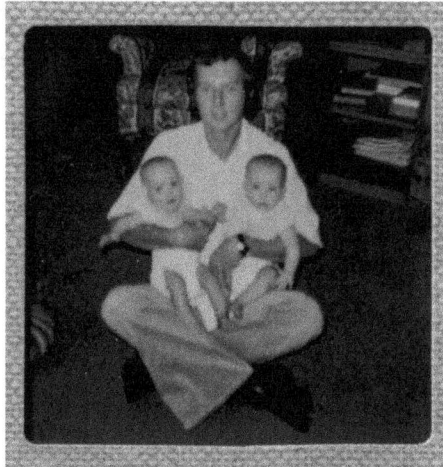

DAD AND DAUGHTERS – Tony Smith holds his twins, Tonya and Toni. He died of a drug overdose at the age of 24 when the girls were 6. (Contributed photo)

not know she was experiencing withdrawal. She just knew she did not want to feel that way. When she told her doctor, he prescribed a drug he said was not addictive.

That was in the 1990s. Today, warnings for the medication, a combination of pentazocine and naloxone, say the narcotic carries a high risk of addiction or dependence.

Over time, Tonya was no longer taking just the prescribed two or three pills a day; she was taking 12-15. Over the years, she needed numerous surgeries, which meant more prescriptions, more pain pills. When she wanted more, she went "doctor shopping." It was easy to game the system then with no central database for pharmacies or doctors to check prescription records.

"I tried to keep it hidden, and I did, for almost 12 years," Tonya says. "I was functional. I was fully aware I had to have the drug to feel normal. I would try to quit. I would try to cut back on my own, but I couldn't."

Her addiction spiraled out of control after her husband – her high school sweetheart – told her he wanted a divorce.

"It made my addiction even worse," she says. "My self-worth was so bad that's what made it really just get in the driver's seat and start driving, and I was no longer in the seat. I wasn't driving, I was just a mere passenger. A runaway train. 'Cause it controls itself.

"I mean you can't, you can't help it. You just … you can't. When you want it, you want it."

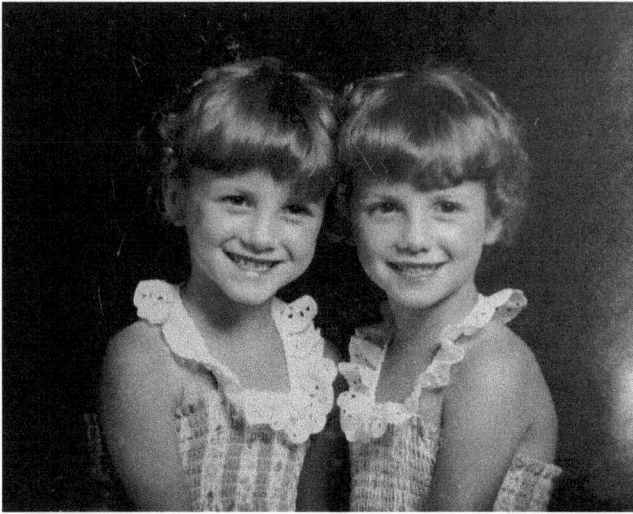

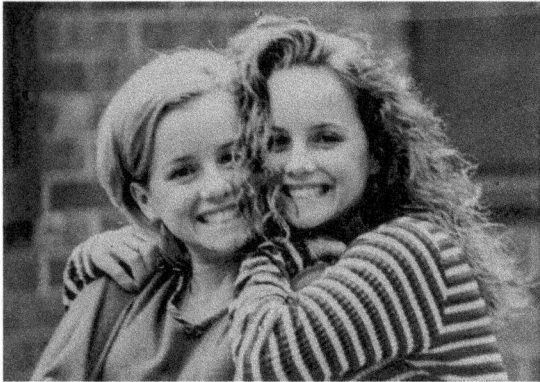

WHO'S WHO? – Tonya and Toni Shinn enjoyed fooling people who could not tell them apart, including teachers and even a boyfriend once. In the top photo, Tonya is on the left; in the bottom picture, she is on the right. (Contributed photos)

'I hated myself'

When she and her husband split, Tonya was 38. She had never lived on her own and was scared. She felt like damaged goods, worthless, no good to anyone.

She started drinking. A lot. Her preferred beverage was vodka. By the time she crashed and burned, she was drinking a gallon-and-a-half of vodka every day. She also popped pills, opiates and tranquilizers, whatever she could get.

Tonya says she did what she could so she and her daughter, a young teen at the time, could get by, but that was not much, and became less and less over time. She pushed everyone else away.

"I didn't do anything but use. I hated myself for what I had become – and for what I felt I had let myself become. I felt like I had dug a hole, dug myself a great big hole and threw the shovel away, and I didn't know how to get out."

For two years, she did not look in a mirror because when she did, she saw a monster. Day after day, she sat on the couch, drinking and swallowing pills. She rarely bathed; that took time away from getting wasted. One day, her sister came over, dragged her to the bathroom and threw her into the shower. Toni repeatedly told her, "I miss my twin."

But an inner voice, Tonya's addiction, talked to her, too. "It talks to you and tells you you're worthless. You're a piece of crap. It wants to kill you."

One morning when she was blind drunk and stoned from drugs, Tonya went into her bedroom closet with her 12-gauge shotgun and closed the door. She planned to end the pain.

"I really felt like my daughter would be better off without me, and so would society," she says. "I couldn't hate myself any more than I did."

Tonya had grown up shooting guns and had shot this one recently. She had cleaned it and put it away. But on this day, with her dog by her side, when she placed the end of the barrel beneath her chin and pulled the trigger, the gun did not fire.

"I kept pulling it, and pulling the trigger," she says, "and I got so angry 'cause I couldn't even kill myself right."

'My sister saved me'

The unsuccessful suicide attempt did not change anything. "I just wanted to hurt me," Tonya says. "I didn't want to hurt anybody else."

She continued to "hurt" herself for a while longer, drinking and drugging herself into oblivion every day. The last day she abused drugs was July 26, 2013. That was the day she overdosed.

"My sister saved me," she says.

That day, Toni told her daughter, Abigail, that she just felt "in her gut" that something was not right. She drove to Tonya's house and found her comatose on the couch.

Many hours later, when she was lucid enough to talk, a doctor at the hospital told Tonya that she should be dead. She weighed just 84 pounds. Her blood alcohol content (BAC) was .48; a BAC of .35 to .40 is potentially fatal.

He asked if she wanted help. She said yes.

A new Tonya

First, she went through detox, six terrible days strapped to a bed at Randolph Hospital. During the entire 3.5-hour ride to a

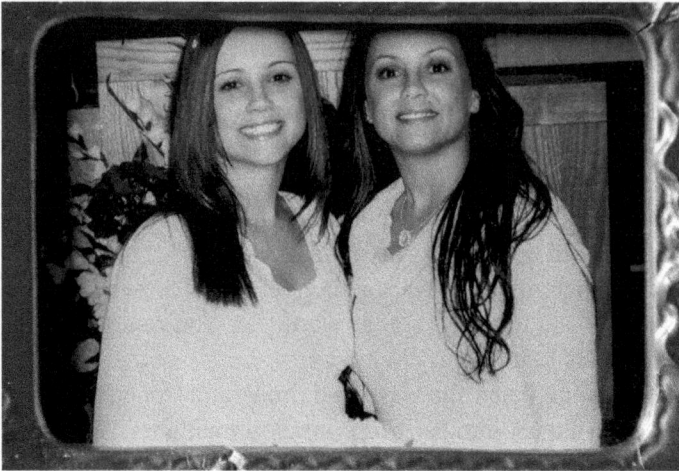

SMILING SISTERS – Tonya Waugh, right, and her twin, Toni Smith, stood up for each other and remained best friends after they each got married. (Contributed photo)

treatment center in Virginia, Tonya cried. She did not know what to expect. She was terrified.

"They said I looked like a broken little bird when I came in there," she says.

She quickly discovered that the people in treatment had walked similar paths and faced similar struggles. She quickly embraced the chance to change.

Fourteen days into the 28-day program, a counselor told her that insurance coverage had hit its limit. She would have to leave the program unless she could cover the balance of her bill. She couldn't. Her ex-husband drove to Virginia the next day and paid $5,600, so she could stay. She says it saved her life.

Her withdrawal from the alcohol and drugs she had depended on for so many years was excruciating. For a time, she felt like spiders were crawling all over her. She threw up so much, and so violently, she developed a hernia. But she only missed one class in 28 days. She knew she would get sick when she went, so she sat next to a trashcan.

After treatment, she relied on faith to see her through. When she felt the urge to use, she prayed and practiced self-love, patience, compassion, understanding.

She calls her addiction the best thing that ever happened to her because in treatment she had to look deep inside and deal with what she found.

"I learned about Tonya, and I came to terms with my past and things that happened. And when I got down to the nitty-gritty dirt in the very bottom of my belly, and knew why I was using, that's when I got better. You have to know why. You've got to get down there and know why. It's ugly. It's angry. It's gross.

"But you face it because that's the only way to get through it. If you don't face it, and go through it, you'll never get around it."

She says it is not willpower alone that keeps her clean and sober: It is knowing Tonya. Liking Tonya. Loving Tonya.

"A new Tonya was born in the mountains. The old one really died. I'm not the same person as I used to be."

Missing Toni

She is not sure when buried wounds from the past and personal problems began to take a toll on her sister. As Tonya had, Toni tried to hide her drinking and drug use. But Tonya knew.

"Hers was really off and on," she says. "It was really after I got clean that Toni's got bad."

On Christmas Eve 2014, Tonya had an unmistakable intuition that something was wrong with Toni – just like Toni had a year earlier when Tonya overdosed. She called Toni's ex-husband, and they each rushed to Toni's house. Tonya's gut feeling had been right. This

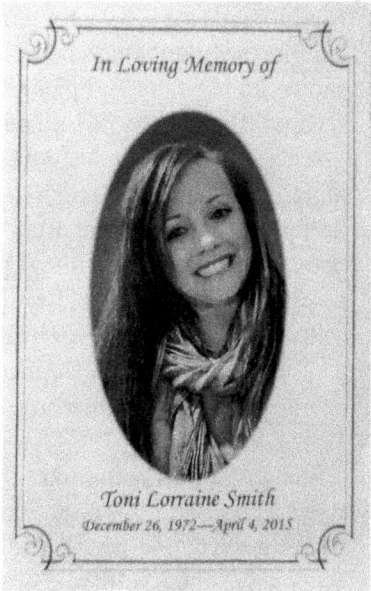

In Loving Memory of

Toni Lorraine Smith
December 26, 1972—April 4, 2015

Toni Lorraine Smith,1972-2015

time, Tonya was the twin who saved her sister's life.

Toni spent Christmas and the twins' 42nd birthday in the hospital. She went from there to in-patient treatment. Tonya says Toni seemed to be doing well after treatment. But 100 days after her Christmas Eve overdose on cocaine, Toni overdosed on methadone – a medication that is used to help wean people off opioids. She died on April 4, 2015.

Tonya spoke and sang at Toni's funeral. She was sorely tempted to break her sobriety, to numb her crushing grief and pain. And then she found herself with a bottle of alcohol. She found it in her house.

"And I sat there with it on my lap. It was a bottle of tequila. I smelled it. For three hours I sat and held it. And I talked to it.

And I told it to get where it needed to go. And that I was done. 'Cause I said I'll show you how much I'm in control here. You're gonna sit right there, and you ain't going nowhere 'til I tell you. And I dumped it out."

Sharing hope

Tonya has found a calling from the wreckage of so many lost years. She says she is also speaking for her sister who no longer has a voice when she shares her story at Narcotics Anonymous meetings, treatment centers, wherever she gets a chance.

"I said from that moment when I went to treatment, this was what I want to do. I've got to return this favor and help those that are like me and that are behind me. I need to put my hand down and reach for them and pick them up."

Hope, she says, is the greatest gift she can give.

After Toni died, Tonya developed bleeding ulcers. A few months ago, she was diagnosed with multiple sclerosis and is living with seizures that often leave her with bruises all over her body. She faces it all without pain medication – she says she has no choice – and tries not to focus on own her trials.

She wants to be the best Tonya she can be, the best mom she can be to her daughter, Kennedy, who is 21, and the best aunt she can be to Toni's daughter, Abigail, who is 19.

Poetic healing

She wrote poems in high school. After Toni died, she wanted to write a poem to read at the funeral, but no words would come. A year later, when inspiration finally came, the floodgates opened. Since then, she has filled many notebooks.

Everything she writes about is from her life, shining a light on the good and the bad. "It made me dig deeper into me," she says. "It's healing me. The more I talk about it, it keeps the monster in that cage."

From a Hopeless Dope Fiend
to a Dopeless Hope Fiend

by Tonya Waugh

Welcome to hell was on the doormat.
Welcome to the worst pain you've ever been in; it should've
said that.
It takes your heart, your soul, and body. Those were the first
three sacrifices.
Then it makes you forget how great your life is.
Or rather, how great your life was before the first three
sacrifices.
Your identity and hope are next on his list.
It rattles the cage, and you take the key out of your pocket.
Now the monster is out of its cage.
Now the monster is ready to rage.
It licks his lips, devouring you entirely; it consumed me.
Like a boxer in the ring ready to fight,
I'm knocking out everyone at first sight.
I hit the ground running.
I'm dodging, I'm ducking.
I kinda like this numb I'm feeling all over me.
This isn't so bad, he says, just wait and see.
Oh, no!! Now I'm completely lost! Those promises were all
lies!!
He said to me, say your last goodbye.

Just for today
Sherri Peery came 'clean' after more than 35 years

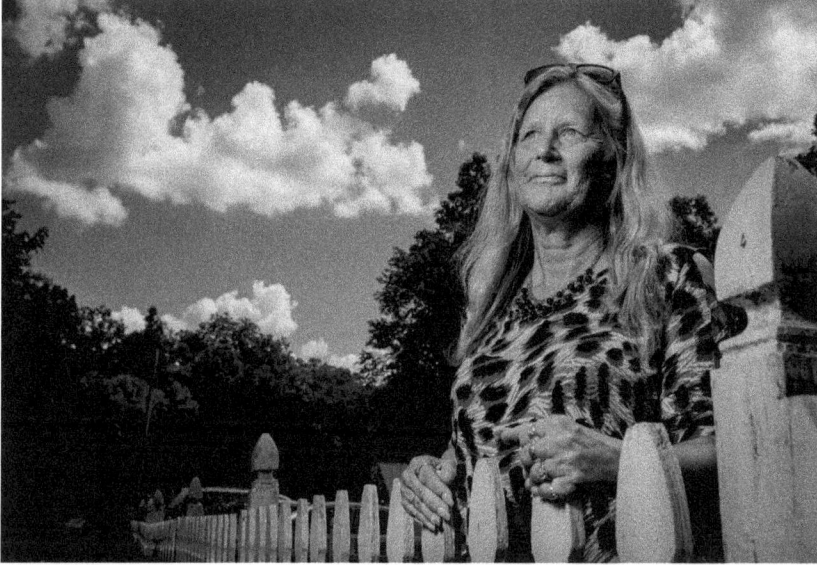

HAPPY DAYS – Sherri Peery plans to celebrate seven years drug-free in October 2019. For 35 years, Peery used and abused a variety of drugs, from alcohol to pain pills. (Photograph by Paul Church/Courtesy The Courier-Tribune)

From the ages of 13 to 49, Sherri Peery abused every drug she could get her hands on.

She had barely entered her teens when she started drinking beer. Smoking marijuana, stolen from her parents' stash, soon followed. In her quest for a high, this California girl who just wanted to have fun tried powder cocaine, acid, angel dust, mushrooms, and crystal meth. The crushing destruction of chasing prescription pills, heroin, and crack came years later.

But Peery always worked, sometimes more than one job, even on the roller coaster ride of using drugs until – decades into her addictions – the overdose deaths of her best friend and her boyfriend within hours of each other sent her into a dangerous, downward spiral.

She wound up on unemployment, with the monthly check

going to her drug dealer. He paid her bills so she could stay in her apartment. Neighbors used her place to package crack cocaine. She sold heroin to pay for the heroin she needed to forget the real world.

Peery finally realized that, without help, drugs were going to kill her. She called her father, and he came to her rescue. She got into treatment somehow and managed to stay clean for more than a year. Then came a relationship with a man who was also in recovery.

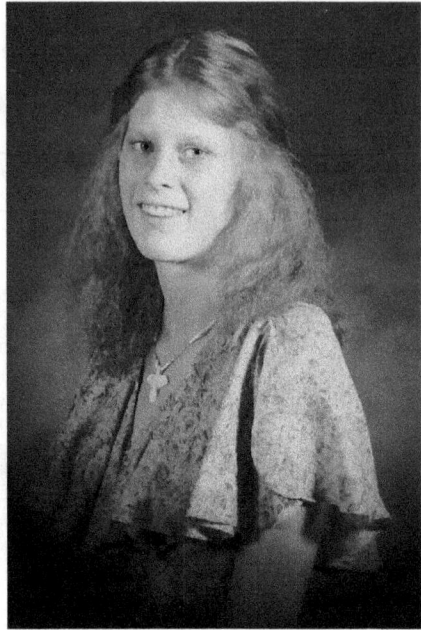
Sherri in high school

When he relapsed, she went searching for him in a crack house. She was high before she found him.

This story probably should not have a happy ending. Against the odds, it does.

Today, Peery has a bachelor's degree in psychology she earned after ditching drugs and is pursuing a master's in mental health counseling with a focus on addiction. She is a residential worker at a Greensboro residential treatment facility. "A lot of the clients tell me," she says, "'I would have never made it without you.'"

And she looks forward to Oct. 3, 2019, when she plans to celebrate seven years of being clean and sober.

A 'functioning' alcoholic, addict

When she was young, Peery said, her father was an abusive drunk who beat her mother and older brother. She recalls that he found religion in jail after being arrested when she was about 10 – and stopped drinking – not long before her partying days began.

She often got into trouble for sneaking out of the house, but harsh discipline did not stop her. She got married a week after she turned 18. She and her husband set up house and devoted their time to "playing hippies" – drinking, smoking marijuana, and using LSD. They had been married for three years when he was killed in a car wreck.

"That's kind of where my life went really bad," she said.

She started drinking heavily and took a job at a biker bar. She said access to a $15,000 insurance settlement from her husband's death nearly killed her. She fell into what she calls a "promiscuous biker life" – drinking, freebasing cocaine, and using the hallucinogenic PCP, also known as angel dust.

After she was raped at a motorcycle rally, she moved back home with her parents. She quit drinking and attended Alcoholics Anonymous meetings. She was sober for about a year, then went to a Grateful Dead concert, where she smoked pot and dropped acid. "It was on," she said.

Eventually, she got a good job and bought a condo. She drank on lunch breaks and used crystal meth, which she also sold on the side, but maintained an appearance of doing, and being, well.

"I was a functioning person in society who was an alcoholic and a drug addict."

A fresh start

Peery drifted in and out of relationships. Then she decided she wanted a baby – someone, in her way of thinking, she would be able to share life with going forward. But she did not want a husband to go with a baby.

She picked a partner because she liked his features. She told the man if she got pregnant it would be the end of the relationship. He did not think she was serious, but when she got pregnant, she sent him packing.

After a baby she named Melody was born in 1989, Peery continued her dual life, working full-time and doing (and selling) drugs part-time. She took Melody to Grateful Dead shows with her. "I thought my life was beautiful," she said.

A close call with the law – she got caught with crystal meth in her car, but a friend claimed it was his – sent her packing to North Carolina when her daughter was about 3. Her parents owned property with cabins, which had once been part of a Boy Scout camp, on Polecat Creek near Randleman. They had bought it because her mother was from the area, and they visited family regularly.

Soon, Peery had taken a job at an Asheboro furniture factory and later secured an apartment in town. She worked hard. She also enrolled at Randolph Community College and worked toward an associate degree in office systems technology.

"My kid was like my motivator," she said. "We were doing

really good, I thought."

But she was not doing "good." She was drinking and doing whatever drugs she could get her hands on, including crystal meth. She had arranged for a girlfriend in California to send it to her by mail.

During the week, Peery worked. On weekends, she partied.

Then came crack

After being charged with driving drunk, Peery quit drinking and started attending Narcotics Anonymous meetings. She met a new beau, and they moved in together.

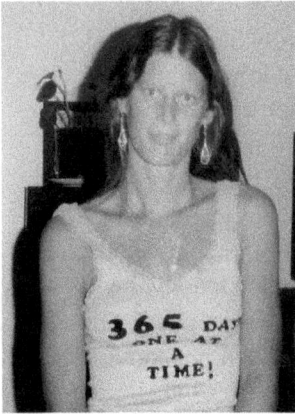

SOBER DRUG USER – Sherri stopped drinking for a year but still was using crystal meth. (Contributed photo)

They smoked a lot of pot. She was selling a lot of it, too. "I was a pretty big weed dealer around here," she said. One day she and her boyfriend of about two years had a fight. He left, and she

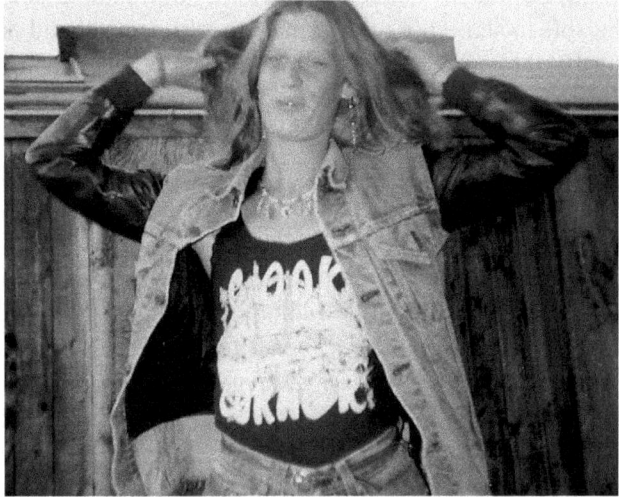

WILD CHILD – Sherri, the California biker girl, poses for a snapshot. (Contributed photo)

never saw him alive again. His body was found in a deer stand 10 days later. He had killed himself.

She fell into a relationship with her boyfriend's best friend, and the drug merry-go-round continued. She split up with him after a failed attempt to get clean, only to get involved with yet another drug user. "I was his weed person," she said. "He was my pill guy."

She did not drink much – because she knew she had a drinking problem – but she smoked a lot of weed and took a lot of prescription pills. She liked the energy she felt after popping whatever pill she could get on the street – and they were plentiful in those days.

Peery was already working full-time when she bought a house in the city and took a second job at a convenience store around the corner. Melody was in her early teens.

A regular in the store told Peery he had something for her one day. He left the store and when he returned, he handed her some crack, a highly concentrated form of cocaine. She was insulted that the fellow thought she'd be interested. But later, she went into a back room and took a few hits. She says she was hooked.

Before long she was stealing from the cash register to support the habit. She was fired when the drawer was $300 short one day.

"That stuff right there, I just wanted it more and more and more. I was ashamed that something had control of me like that."

Shooting up

She was still doing crack and pills when she landed a job at a music club near the Randolph/Guilford county line. "I couldn't stop," she said.

Things got so bad eventually that she owed her crack dealer her entire check when she got paid. She couldn't pay her bills. Her house was in foreclosure. Her car was repossessed.

When she told her boyfriend about her crack problem, he accused her of having an affair with the dealer. "I really was (having an affair)," she said. "It was just with the pipe." When she admitted her crack problem to her daughter, Melody packed and moved to her grandparents' house.

Once again, Peery tried getting clean again. This was the fourth time. She started attending NA, but just could not shake the crack. She picked up a chip signifying she had not used in 30 days even though that was not true.

Her family believed her. Her daughter moved back home. Her father and brothers helped keep her from losing her house.

"I promised them I was going to stop, but I couldn't. That crack cocaine had my head so spinning that all I could think of was calling that dude" who supplied it.

After two months, Melody left again. Peery and her boyfriend split, then got back together and moved to Greensboro. They were running from the drugs, the lies, the money troubles.

Of course, they took all their woes with them. For the next three years, they lived in a motel. She had a job; his contribution to their income was "boosting," which is what drug users call shoplifting.

Most of their money went to buy heroin because it was cheap. Peery recalls being angry the day she discovered her boyfriend had started shooting up heroin, instead of snorting the powder. Her response was to get someone to shoot her up, too.

She had always told herself that at least her addiction was not as bad as that of the people who injected drugs. And, just like that, she was one of them.

'I was lost'

Peery's parents cut contact when they learned of this new low, but that did not change anything. In March 2010, she and her boyfriend moved into a small apartment. A couple of days later, she got a call that a very good friend had died.

Her boyfriend got home from a day of boosting as she was leaving to go to visit her friend's parents. He asked if she wanted him to go, too. She told him, no, that she would see him later.

When she returned that evening, she thought he was passed out, but he was dead from an overdose.

"I lost my best friend and my boyfriend hours apart," she said. "I was lost. I was 100 percent lost."

Peery opened her apartment to anyone who had drugs and spiraled even further into a pit of drug abuse. "I don't know how I didn't die then – I really don't. I called my mama a couple of times, but she wasn't ready to talk to me. My dad came to take me to eat – probably the only time I ate."

The day she called her father and pleaded with him to come get her the next morning, he was knocking on her door at 6 a.m. He wondered why she was not packed. "I was so incapable; I couldn't do anything. I waited for my dad to come."

He took her to a hospital, where she told the staff she would die if they did not help her get help. Somehow, she said, she wound up at an addiction treatment center, where she detoxed and completed a two-week program.

"It was the first time I heard, 'You have a disease. You don't have a drug problem. You have a disease.'"

She spent time at a couple of halfway houses and found a job at a telephone center in Greensboro.

Relapse – again

Everything was good for about a year. Then she met a guy.

"He relapsed, and I went to the crack house to try to find him, but before I could find him, I was high again."

Peery immediately regretted her relapse. She called her NA sponsor, who went with her to tell her family what had happened. "My daughter said, 'Never call me again.' I couldn't blame her."

It shook her to her core to watch her father remove the one-year chip she had given him – the token that signified she had been clean and sober for a year – from his keyring.

She did not want to use again but did not know what else to do. Her family wanted nothing to do with her, and her "friends" had heroin. During this relapse, she turned to prostitution so she could pay for her next high.

Eventually, she called on her father once again and entered treatment once again. When she was released, she was terrified of the potential for using drugs again, so she boarded a bus and left her familiar surroundings behind. She traveled to Iowa, where a girlfriend she had known since they were preschoolers, was living. The time was good for her, she said, but by Christmas she wanted to return home.

The folks at home were not ready for her. In March, she asked again, and they said yes.

Reconnection

Within a month, Peery had found work at an Asheboro manufacturing plant and had returned to school. In Iowa, she had started working a 12-step program she had never taken seriously before. Back in North Carolina, she continued that path.

When she celebrated her first year of sobriety, her parents were at the meeting, but not her daughter. Her parents came when she marked two years, too, but her daughter still was not speaking to her. On the third anniversary of her clean date, her daughter showed up. Everyone in the room was in tears.

Her daughter still was not ready to resume their relationship. That took years. Then one day Melody, who had a 7-year-old and a 6-month-old baby, called Peery. She asked if Peery was home, and then, to someone on her end of the line, asked, "What are you going to do?" Then the call was disconnected.

When Melody would not answer return calls, a frantic Peery dialed 911. She learned that her daughter's boyfriend had assaulted her with a baseball bat, and she had taken refuge at a neighbor's house; an ambulance was on the way.

While Melody healed – she had suffered a concussion, two broken arms, and needed 17 staples to close the wounds in her scalp – Peery took a leave of absence from work to care for her and her two young granddaughters.

Today, Peery says she and her daughter "have been like peas and carrots ever since." She sometimes takes her granddaughters with her to 12-step meetings. When those with a year or more of clean time are asked to raise their hands, Peery, of course, raises her. So does Ava, her older granddaughter, who is 4.

'Love-hate' relationship

Peery took a sizeable pay cut and added about 30 minutes to her commute when she took her current job at a substance abuse treatment center.

The work is important to her. It is important to the work that she has intimate knowledge of the doubts and fears the people she interacts with are going through.

Sometimes people who have just arrived at the treatment facility are having second thoughts. She understands. The thought of trying to quit using drugs forever can be nauseating and paralyzing at the same time.

"It's scary when you say, 'I'm going to stop' doing something. It's breaking up with your best friend. It's a love-hate relationship for sure."

"When you're in early recovery that seems impossible. After they get through a couple of days, and their mind clears up a little bit, they start getting some hope back – because you are hopeless."

She tells people in early recovery something those with years of clean time understand: They do not need to contemplate years, months, or even weeks of abstinence.

They need to focus on remaining drug-free for a much shorter, and more manageable, length of time: Just for today.

'I shouldn't be where I am'

Scott Smith, convicted felon at 18, is clean, sober, and gainfully employed

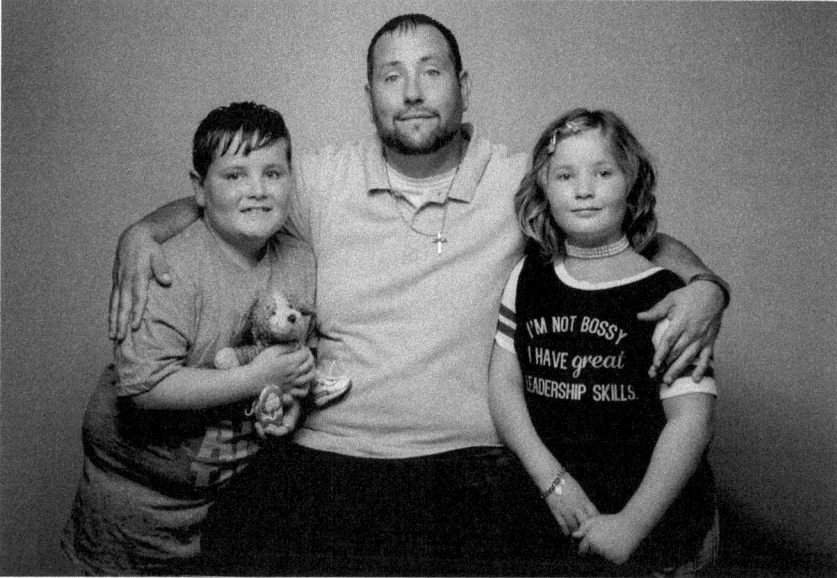

FATHER AND HIS TWINS – Scott Smith proudly sat for a portrait with his twins, Eva and Avery. They started third grade this year. (Photograph by Paul Church/ Courtesy The Courier-Tribune)

These two stories by Chip Womick appeared in The (Asheboro, N.C.) Courier-Tribune, the first one in 2018, the second in 2014. They are reprinted with permission.

This is what goes through Scott Smith's mind when he thinks about the opioid epidemic: "By God's grace, that's not me."

Smith, who is 40, lives in Asheboro. He was an active addict for more than a decade, but he has not used illegal drugs or used legal drugs illegally – both of which were once part of his everyday existence – for more than six years.

He credits God – and methadone – with saving his life.

A couple of years after he landed a spot in a Greensboro methadone clinic, where he drove daily for a dose of the drug

69

that quelled the cravings and withdrawal symptoms, he found a job despite a felony conviction on his record.

He said he is grateful to Easter Seals UCP North Carolina for giving him that chance. He worked as a peer support specialist, using his life experience to help others on the road to recovery.

Today, he works for another agency, helping people with serious mental illnesses (who qualify) get the support they need to live independently.

He's been off methadone for years. Now he takes Suboxone daily to quell his anxiety while it keeps opioid cravings at bay. If he needs to take the drug for the rest of his life, that's OK by him.

He is a high school dropout (who earned a GED) with a significantly checkered past, yet he has a good-paying job.

And he is clean and sober.

"I shouldn't be where I am without God's help," he said. "I feel like we all owe a debt of gratitude to God. Maybe mine's a little greater than yours."

Ditching drugs

A year or two before he got a spot in the program at a Greensboro methadone clinic, Smith tried quitting "cold turkey" – detoxing for a week and then spending another two weeks in an in-patient facility.

He continued to feel bad due to withdrawal. Six months later, he relapsed.

Based on his experience, Smith believes most long-time opioid abusers will need medication to help beat their addiction.

"I don't know any other way anybody's going to get off opiates," he said. "If you are a person that gets extremely 'dopesick' when you don't have it, it's not going to work."

Everyone does not experience the same withdrawal symptoms. One of Smith's was a spike in his temperature to 101 or higher; he said he's never heard of anyone else who experienced that.

But there were plenty of other symptoms: Dizziness, headache, cold sweats, hot sweats, shaking, diarrhea and whole-body pain.

"If I woke up and didn't have something to put in my arm or up my nose, within an hour I'd be in serious withdrawal. It's probably the most miserable you can be without being physically injured or being on your deathbed."

Smith noted that, where it is legal, medical marijuana is being used to wean people off opiates, a treatment he calls "much safer than Suboxone or methadone."

The epidemic

Many opioid pill abusers switch to heroin when prescriptions become hard to get. Heroin is also cheaper. But heroin is often cut with fentanyl, a synthetic opioid that is about 100 times stronger than morphine. Fentanyl-laced heroin use leads to deadly overdoses.

Smith recalls switching back to pills from heroin because he knew exactly what he was getting in the pills. And while opioids are grabbing headlines these days, he said another drug should be in the news, too: Methamphetamine.

"Right now the biggest problem is meth ... Everybody that I know that had made an attempt to get off opiates, they are shooting meth like they were shooting heroin. Meth is the worst drug ever."

* * *

This story by Chip Womick first appeared in The (Asheboro) Courier-Tribune in 2014. It is reprinted with permission.

A few months' back – and for the first time in years – Scott Smith began to feel like somebody.

The new perception he has of himself comes from a new job with Easter Seals UCP North Carolina.

He is a peer support specialist – that is, someone living in recovery with mental illness or a substance abuse disorder who provides support to individuals who can benefit from their experiences.

It's a real job, helping real people.

"Until I started doing this, I felt completely invisible," Smith said in a recent interview, "and now I'm starting to feel more visible."

Smith, who is 35, had almost given up on ever getting a chance at such a job.

Or on being "visible."

Doing drugs, laying low

He has spent a good portion of his life doing drugs and says he was "a functioning addict" for about a decade. He has smoked, swallowed and shot up a laundry list of substances, from pot to opium.

He dropped out of high school his junior year, but later got his GED through RCC.

At 18, he was a convicted felon.

His conviction on charges of larceny and possession of stolen goods stemmed from a night smoking crack cocaine when he was 17. He had met an older fellow at a friend's house and they partied all night. For fun, they threw rocks at each other. After passing out in a car parked

71

in a town park, they woke up and returned to the friend's house, where the older man started taking stuff.

Smith was scared of the man. He joined in.

He was married, then divorced in his early 20s. Another relationship ended when a woman who was carrying his child left him after finding a syringe in the home they shared.

She knew he popped pills, he said, but thought he was using the syringe to shoot up. The needle belonged to a friend, Smith said; he did not graduate to shooting up for a few years.

The father of five, he has no contact with three of his children.

He has held a succession of jobs, but also has lost, or left, a succession of jobs.

He has stolen things to support his habit.

And, at one time, nearly everyone near and dear had given up on him.

All because of illegal – or illegally used – drugs.

A felony record does not look good on a job application. Over the years, he often could not find work that paid above minimum wage due to his checkered past.

"It was like I was totally invisible," Smith said. "I could not find a job."

He admits that there also were times when he wanted to fly beneath the radar, so he could use and sell drugs – he says he once made $1,500 a week selling marijuana – without attracting the attention of lawmen or the tax man.

"I had to be kind of invisible," he said. "I had money. I couldn't use it to do flashy (things) so I would stay home and get high."

There also were times when the rest of the world was largely invisible to him.

"I wanted it to be that way," he said, "because I was probably trying to figure out a way to screw them over."

A chance to change

The last time he was busted he was 32. He and his girlfriend were living in a motel in Alamance County. Their primary pastime was shooting up heroin.

One morning after they had been up all night getting high there was a knock at their room door. Smith opened it to find two officers.

Later, they moved back to Randolph County. They had two babies; the water and power had been turned off in their trailer and they were on the verge of being evicted. But they were still doing drugs.

Smith said his mother – and most everyone else who might have come to his assistance – had given up on him. An aunt stepped up with the reminder that he was family and worth another shot.

"If it wasn't for her, I would not be clean to this day," he said.

His current life bears no resemblance to his former one.

Things changed when he and his girlfriend landed a spot in a Greensboro methadone clinic. They drive to the clinic from Asheboro every morning to get a dose of methadone.

Methadone clinics help wean people dependent on heroin or prescription pain pills off the drugs.

In the beginning, he received a minuscule dosage. The amount was increased gradually to nearly 100 milligrams a day, before a gradual decrease began. He is down to 40 mg daily and hopes to stop taking methadone altogether in about six months.

The clinic, he said, saved his life.

'Got to start somewhere'

He has been "clean" – meaning that he has not used any illegal drugs – for almost two years and is confident he can maintain that sobriety.

"I'm very proud of that, obviously," he said. "I don't ever want to feel that again."

Yet, he says, for the most part, he would not change his experience of addiction.

"I've done a lot of things I feel bad about," he said, "but I never molested children. I haven't killed nobody."

He sees his survival of a checkered past as what helped land him his job as a peer support specialist because he has experience and hope to share. He plans to make the most of his chance.

"When you help people, you start to help yourself and you start to feel visible and part of the community again," he said. "... I feel like I'm part of something, a greater good, something that can make a difference.

"Not worldwide, but just to one person. I mean everybody would like to make a difference worldwide, I guess. You just got to start somewhere.

"And even if you can just make one person feel better, do better, or be better, you've accomplished something and you're a part of something, and you're definitely a visible person at that point."

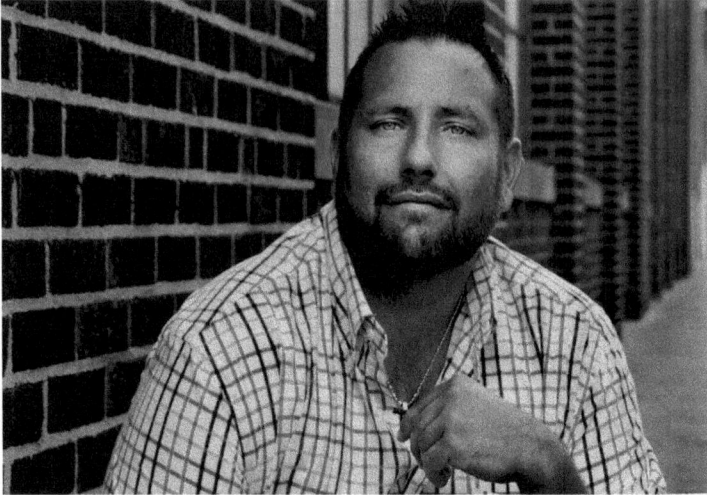

Scott Smith poses in 2015. (Paul Church/Courtesy The Courier-Tribune)

What Scott says ...

My name is David Scott Smith. I was addicted to opiates until 2012, and this is an update on what has happened since the last story in The Courier-Tribune. I have had custody of my twins, Eva and Avery Smith, for a little over two years. They attend Guy B. Teachey Elementary School and are in the third grade. It has been difficult being a single dad who has paid child support for three other children and is still paying for one.

We have a small but loyal circle of family and friends. My children and I attend church, as well as the NETworX for Hope Randolph group that is faith-based. I realized God has kept me here for a reason, and, as long as my children and I keep God first, we will come out the other side of any struggle.

I lost one of my best friends on May 3, 2019, to an overdose – and an estranged cousin to the same fate due to opiates.

I have become a recognized call-in character on the 2 Guys Named Chris Show on Rock 92 radio. I call myself "Heroin Scott." It gives me a platform to talk about the disease and to laugh at it, which, for me, takes power away from the disease. I would love to have a bigger stage to discuss and shed more light on addiction and recovery.

Last, but most important, I want to thank God for the grace and forgiveness he has granted me. Love God above all else and your neighbor as you love yourself.

'People do change'
Amber Mabe wants to help others overcome addiction too

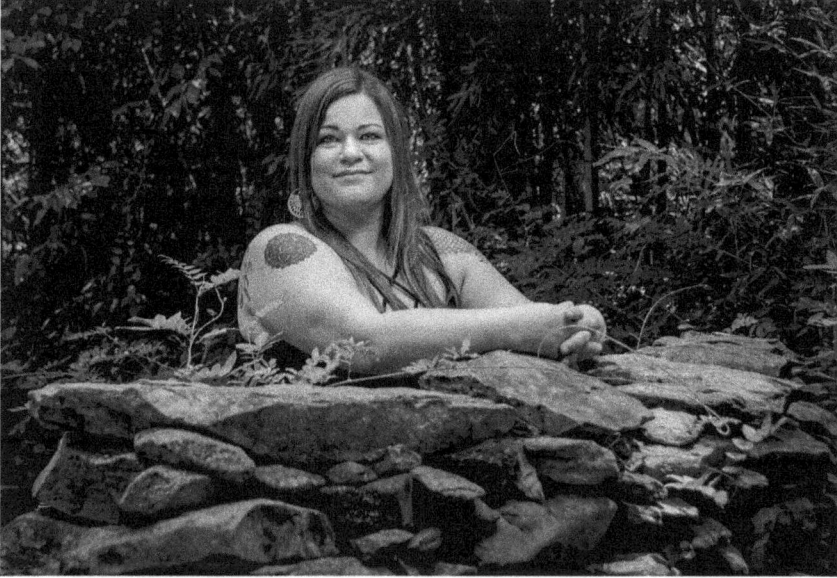

FIRST CAME A PRESCRIPTION – Amber Mabe struggled to stop abusing drugs
for nearly five years. Her greatest challenge was quitting methamphetamines.
(Photograph by Paul Church/Courtesy The Courier-Tribune)

Amber Mabe was almost 30 before she plunged into a rabbit hole of drug use – opiates, then methamphetamines – that cratered her life.

She lost her children. She lost her business. She lost herself.

In the darkest days, she and her husband (now her ex-husband) stole from stores to finance the next round of drugs. In the beginning, she stayed outside to drive the getaway car. Later she joined him because two people can steal more.

Eventually, they got caught, and she still faces a day in court on those charges. She has watched store surveillance video that shows her in the act of shoplifting.

"I can't even wrap my brain around it now," she says. "It's embarrassing, and it just makes me cringe, but it is what it is, and, of course, I've learned from it. I wasn't raised to steal. I was not a thief or anything like that prior to drugs.

75

"It's just a … it really made me act like a different person. Not so much the substances themself, but the desire to have more of it."

Mabe spent about five years in and out of active addiction. Every time she stopped using, she fell back into the pit, lured by a powerful psychological pull she cannot explain.

She quit for what she's confident will be the last time on March 2, 2019.

"I don't want to go back to where I was just a few months ago," she says, "living in my vehicle and not having a job and just struggling to find the will to keep living."

Drugs for this and that

Mabe was so shy in school that when the teacher called her name she could hardly think; if she had to stand in front of the class, she froze. Students teased her. A school counselor suggested therapy; she started that at 9.

As early as kindergarten, she struggled with body image. She was an early teen when her insecurities led to ping-ponging between anorexia (starving herself to lose weight) and bulimia (gorging and then making herself throw up, also to lose weight). She says she thinks she just wanted to have control over something in her life.

When her parents found out about the bulimia, she went to more therapy and, for a while, took an amphetamine-like drug prescribed to suppress appetite.

In her junior year, when the social scene – the drama, the cliques – got to be too much, she left high school and went to Randolph Community College to get her adult high school diploma. Then she enrolled in RCC's graphic design program, which was a natural fit. She had been drawing and doodling ever since she could remember.

When she recognized that she could focus in class only was when she was drawing and doodling, she again reached out for help. A diagnosis of ADHD (attention deficit hyperactivity disorder) came with a prescription for Adderall, an amphetamine. The pills did not simply calm her down so she could function, as intended; they knocked her out. She did not take them long.

Over the years, she was off and on different antidepressants, trying to find something that made her feel better. What the drugs did best, she says, was lead to weight gain, which made her more depressed. Mabe did not become addicted to the drugs prescribed in her younger days but wonders what role they may have played on her road to addiction.

"I didn't know at the time that I was basically taking something (amphetamines) that I would become addicted to later in another form … There's been so many elements that I think play into the road to addiction for me."

Enter opiates

After graduation, Mabe found a good job in her field. She also opened an online graphics store offering custom logos and branding for small businesses. Sales doubled and then nearly tripled in two or three years. She left her job to be her own boss, with clients from all over the world.

In 2012, she reconnected with a former high school classmate who had moved away from the area for a few years. They started dating in May and married in December. By 2014, they had two sons.

Caring for the children and keeping her business going left little time for sleep. One day she fell asleep at the wheel, and her car ran off the road. A fence and a tree kept the vehicle from plunging into a pond, but her face bounced off the steering wheel. She was not severely injured but left the hospital with a swollen face, two black eyes, and a prescription for a medication that combines two pain relievers – acetaminophen and oxycodone, which is an opioid.

At first, she took the pills as the doctor had ordered. When she noticed that pills were disappearing, she discovered that her husband had been taking them. When they reconnected, he told her that he had battled addiction but was no longer using. He had lied. He had been shooting up drugs the whole time.

When she stopped taking the pain pills, she developed the worst flu-like symptoms she had ever experienced. Her husband told her she was "dopesick" – sick because the body was missing the "dope" to which it had become accustomed. His advice: Take more pills if you don't want to stay sick for days. So, she did.

'This is dumb'

After she found out about her husband's drug use, Mabe was angry, but her displeasure did not change his ways. She could not understand how a drug could be so enticing that he would chase it and neglect her, their children, their life together.

A few weeks after Mabe's accident, her husband brought a mutual friend to their apartment. The woman arrived with needles and Opana, a powerful prescription opioid. Mabe was livid. While she and her husband argued, the woman retreated to the bathroom where – using water, a lighter, and the pills – she prepared a liquid they could inject.

In a moment born of spite and despair, Mabe asked the visitor to shoot her up. If it's good enough for you, it's good enough for me, she told her husband.

Mabe felt nothing from the first injection, so the woman gave her another. This time, she felt a sudden warmth flowing down the back of her neck; then she got dizzy and threw up the rest of the night.

Despite the nausea that always followed, that flush of heat – fleeting relief from tension she perpetually carried in her neck and shoulders – brought Mabe back for more. After a few days of shooting up with her husband, she briefly returned to her senses. "This is dumb," she thought. "This is not what I want to do with my life."

But she had already reached a point of no return. She could not quit without painful withdrawal symptoms. So, she fell into a pattern: Just use enough to prevent being sick. But addiction is not that simple. Before long, the opiates had control.

Trying to quit

Mabe decided to shoot up on her own one day when her husband was not home. She thought she knew how but missed the vein. Within 24 hours she had developed a painful infection.

She called on her mother to drive her to the hospital because her husband did not want to go. She told her mother what was going on -- the first anyone in her family knew of her drug use. Then she told the emergency room physician. She received IV antibiotics in the hospital and was discharged with two prescriptions: an antibiotic and a mild opiate, eight pills that, she was told, would help with withdrawal.

Her first round of addiction lasted about three months. Miserable and determined to kick the habit, she went to a doctor and got a prescription for Suboxone, a medication that lets people wean themselves off stronger narcotics.

Mabe separated from her husband, quit shooting up, tapered off the Suboxone, and was clean for nearly nine months.

"I didn't go to NA (Narcotics Anonymous). I didn't go to any kind of therapy that I needed to. I was just kind of doing everything on my own, which was stupid."

Then her husband called. He had been arrested and wanted her to pay his bond. Thinking of their children – and missing him despite their past – she bailed him out. Being with him triggered the drug demon. "Within an hour," she says, "we were buying a pill."

In 2015, pills were easy to come by. Then, a 40-mg. Opana cost $60 to $80 on the street. Mabe says she has heard that the price is double that now, if not more, because prescription pills are so hard to find due to stricter laws and oversight.

And then came meth

2016 was a very bad year for Mabe. The Department of Social Services entered the picture after her husband got angry and hit her over something she said to her mother while talking to her on the phone.

She went to the hospital; he went to jail; their children, by order of DSS, went to live with Mabe's parents (and still live there).

In the summer of 2016, she shot up methamphetamines for the first time. She knew immediately that the drug was going to be trouble for her. Opiates made her sick; meth made her feel the best she had ever felt.

"I think," she says, "what made it hard for me to walk away from it is that it didn't make me do crazy things like other people."

Hallucinations and delusions are common among meth users. Mabe has watched a woman on meth pick her nose apart with a pair of tweezers because she thought a bug had crawled up it. She has seen a man scamper 60 feet up a tree to hide from police officers who did not exist.

Meth calmed her, made her feel lucid, organized, and, in her mind, normal. Still, she tried to quit. While chasing to repeat the euphoric experience she'd had with meth the first time, she stopped and then relapsed back-to-back-to-back.

She never experienced the intensity of that initial high again. But she did experience more loss: her business, her apartment, her vehicle, most everything except her compulsion to use.

'People do change'

As her addiction waxed and waned, her family grew with the birth of two more boys. Both wound up in foster care. Social Services took her youngest in June of 2018 when he was 6 days old.

"It threw me into the biggest relapse of my life," Mabe says. "I had no will left in me to try to rectify my mistakes."

A few months later she mustered the will and checked into rehab, but only made it for three days. She returned to her husband time after time because she had nowhere else to go; he was living with his mother. When she left him the last time, in February of 2019, she lived in her van.

Mabe spent a month in a halfway house but moved out after one of the other women died of a heroin overdose in the bathroom. She moved to a friend's house for a couple of days before returning to her parents' house.

In August of 2019, she moved into her own apartment for the first time in four years. Her older sons can visit, and while her younger boys remain in

ALL TOGETHER – Amber Mabe was with all of her children – left to right, Lealand, 5, Lyndon, 1, Liam, 6, and Gabe, 2 – for the first time ever in June of 2019. She is working hard to be reunited with her boys. (Contributed photo)

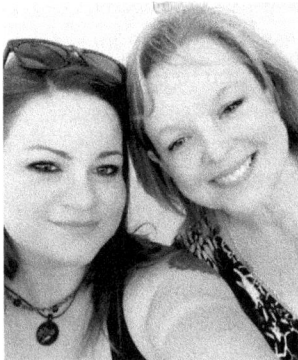

foster care, she has been working diligently on a case plan so that one day she can regain custody.

She has a new job and her own business, Mandowla Creative (www.etsy.com/shop/customlogobrands), is up and running again. She also has new purpose and lessons to share.

"I think that part of my recovery is the cathartic feeling of helping another person and hoping that they get through it like you did."

Perhaps the biggest lesson, she says, is that recovery requires active participation, something she did not understand until a few months ago. She says that's why she failed repeatedly in her attempts to stop abusing drugs.

She attends two or three 12-step meetings every week, where she hears messages that help keep her on the right track and where she has found friends who know what she has been through. She goes to individual therapy and participates in two support groups.

She also has a message for people who have never used drugs: Stigma is another hurdle in recovery – a big one.

"I have seen other people struggle

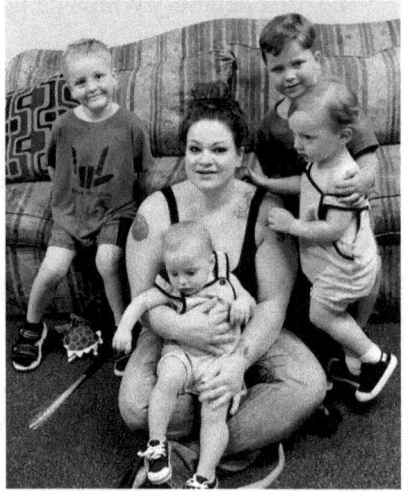

Amber and her mom, Tammy Mabe

and give up and relapse because of being repeatedly turned down for positions that they probably would have done very well in had they been given a chance," she says. "People do change. And they do recover."

'Hell on earth'
Preston Cross found relief from PTSD in alcohol, other drugs

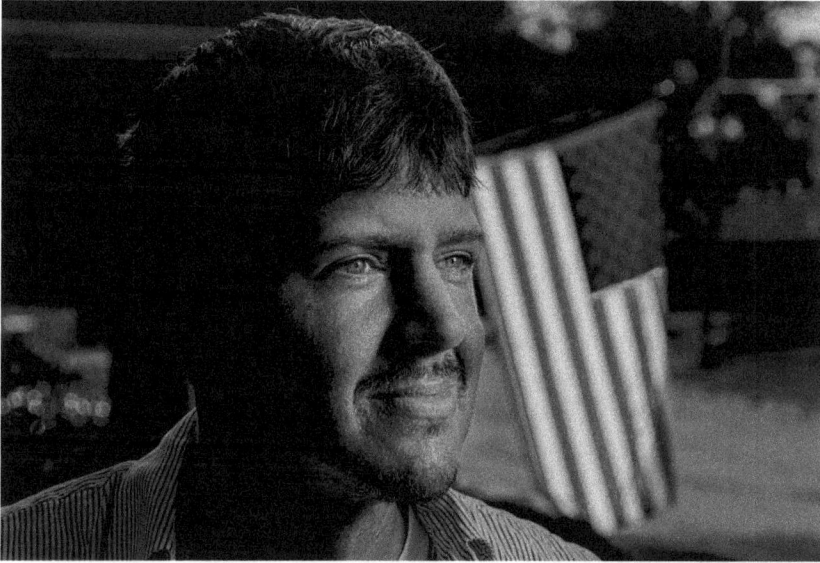

LOST TIME – Preston Cross spent several years drinking before he found harder drugs to mask the pain of memories from his service days in Iraq in 2006 and 2007. (Photograph by Paul Church/Courtesy The Courier-Tribune)

Preston Cross brought his nightmares home from Iraq. The nightmares were the replay from 10 months manning a machine gun on the back of a truck in a war zone. The dreams featured death and destruction, mortar rounds, roadside bombs, and explosions, explosions, explosions.

"Every day of the week I thought I was going to die," Cross says. "Every mission I thought I was going to die."

He did not think he would make it home alive, but, he did. The drinking started immediately: A sip of liquor first thing in the morning to quell the shakes, followed by a day of hard drinking.

Looking for answers to his drinking, anger, and fitful dreams, Cross journeyed in 2008 to the W. G. (Bill) Hefner VA Medical Center in Salisbury. He went to the emergency department but was directed to the mental health clinic where he was told he was suffering from PTSD (post-traumatic stress disorder). He was sent home with prescription drugs. Cross took the pills and kept drinking.

The substance abuse continued – drinking and a brief dalliance with cocaine – until after he received his honorable discharge in 2014. Then, cocaine reemerged, and heroin and pills joined the fray. Anything to dull the memories. Make them go away.

The first time an acquaintance shot cocaine into his veins, Cross marveled and thanked the man. "It was the greatest feeling that I've ever felt in my life," he says. "And that's when I had dedicated my life to nothing but drugs from there on out. I knew I was going to take drug use to my grave."

But he didn't. By his count, Cross has been in a mental hospital 10 or 12 times because he wanted so badly to beat his drug addiction.

"I always went back to rehab. Always went back to intensive outpatient. Always went back to groups. NA meetings. Always went back to the hospital and committed myself. Always, until I figured it out. And it was the hardest thing in my life to do."

In September of 2018, he succeeded. He has been clean and sober for more than a year. His girlfriend is expecting their child. They are financially stable. They have a home. And a dog. He is happier than he has ever been: "I feel like I'm living happily ever after right now."

Cross shares his story to show those still stuck in lives dominated by drugs that there is hope: "If you never give up, eventually you will find that path to recovery. Guaranteed. It's gonna happen."

Eager to join

Cross had wanted to be in the Army since he was a kid. He quit high school his junior year to enlist, then quickly earned his GED at Randolph Community College in Asheboro, so he could qualify for service.

But he failed the hearing test and was told he needed an operation. A year later, after surgery on both ears, he tried again and failed the test again. He thought his dream was not to be.

About a year later, he saw a flier that advertised good jobs burying cable. He called the 800 number, and an Army National Guard recruiter answered. Cross told the man he wanted to join and explained his history and why he could not. The recruiter told him all he needed was a hearing waiver.

Soon, thanks to what he thought was a waiver from the

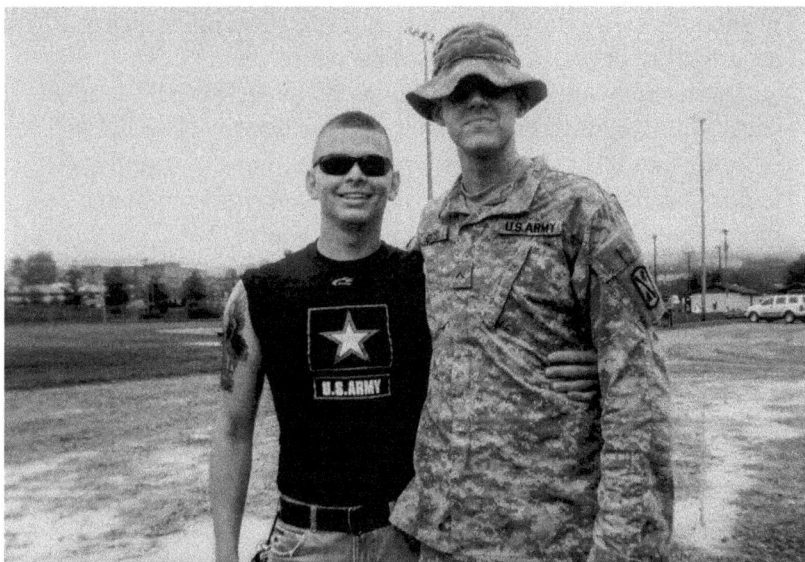

LOST TIME – Preston Cross, right, and his older brother, Roger, each came home from Iraq with post traumatic stress disorder. For years after they returned home, they were 'drug buddies,' constantly looking for drugs to kill their memories. (Contributed photo)

recruiter, Cross took an oath of enlistment in Charlotte. Six weeks into basic training, someone figured out that he did not have a waiver. He was summoned to talk to a captain.

"They say you can't hear," the captain said. "Can you hear me talk?"

Cross said yes.

"Do you want to be here?" the captain asked.

"More than anything," Cross replied.

The captain snapped his fingers and asked if Cross could hear it. Cross said he could hear it "just fine."

"OK, carry on," the captain said. "I'll take care of it."

And he did, never mind that Cross has 70 percent hearing loss in one ear and 80 percent loss in the other.

'We kept it to ourselves'

He loved the Army and his job in field artillery, training at Fort Bragg as a crew member on an M270, an armored, self-propelled, multiple rocket launcher.

On a Wednesday morning in August of 2006 he got a call that he was being reclassified as mounted infantry and transferred to a different unit. Three days later, he was aboard a plane bound for Iraq.

The day after he arrived in Iraq, he received his first lesson in shooting a 240 Bravo machine gun. His new unit provided security for convoys up and down the entire country.

"I was eager," he says. "I couldn't wait to get started. I was 20 years old. I've never seen combat, and I was ready. Two weeks of being into Iraq I was praying to God nothing else would happen, and I was praying up to 30 times a day that nothing more would happen, and I'd make it home alive."

The first experience that shook him was a mortar attack aimed at his truck. His Humvee was the last vehicle in a convoy, and he was facing the rear, his machine gun ready. The convoy stopped because a convoy in front had found an IED (improvised explosive device) that needed to be disarmed.

As soon as the trucks stopped, a mortar exploded about 100 meters behind his vehicle, followed by a hail of bullets aimed his way. Cross returned fire, about 100 rounds in a firefight that lasted about 20 seconds. A second mortar exploded so close behind his truck that it took his breath away. "It made my head fuzzy. It was that close. I felt the heat off of it."

He shot another 250 rounds in a second firefight before getting support from another truck in his unit. No one was hurt, but he was shaken.

"That was one of the first incidents that made me realize what I was really, what I really got myself into, and it was no more fun. It was time for me to really try to make it home."

Later, he was with a convoy crawling slowly through Baghdad in the middle of the night, using spotlights to sweep the road for IEDs, when an explosion rocked the lead truck. Seared into his memory is an image of the gunner's face, half blown away, and the sound of the man screaming that he could not feel his lips.

Firefights were a nightly occurrence on missions. Those he did not mind so much; they brought an adrenaline rush. The roadside bombs and RPGs (rocket-propelled grenades) were a different matter; when they exploded close by, it would take his breath away. Rockets and mortars aimed at the base during "down time" were commonplace. "It's the scariest thing imaginable," he says. "You think you're just going to die any second."

During his tour, he saw fellow soldiers sustain terrible injuries; two died.

Also etched in his memory is the picture of a small Iraqi girl standing by a road in the middle of the desert in the middle of winter. There was no sign of life as far as he could see. He was freezing in top-of-the-line military winter gear. She was wearing only a fluffy pink coat. No pants. No shoes. No hat. No gloves. Cross says he felt an overwhelming sorrow as his convoy moved on.

"Iraq in 2006 was hell on earth. It was a complete nightmare. … The morale was so low; everybody was so down and depressed because we were so tired because we were on missions so often. We never had a day off."

After seeing his fellow gunner injured in the explosion in Baghdad, Cross sought help from the combat stress unit. He was surprised to find that the soldier on duty to counsel him was not much older than he was. He did not find relief. He says he was told to chill out, carry on, and he would be OK. He never went back.

After that, Cross says he accepted the idea that he was going to die. His fear disappeared. He wanted action. He was eager to engage with the enemy. To find somebody to shoot at. Or kill.

Cross says he saw several soldiers "wig out" and threaten suicide. He says that eight soldiers who deployed with him did kill themselves. But no one talked about it.

"Nobody shared anything with anybody. We kept it to ourselves until we got home."

Expensive habit

After he came home, Cross drank a lot. In the beginning, the booze flowed to celebrate getting back together with his older brother, Roger, and his old buddies, but it continued when he was alone.

"I didn't know how to transition," he says. "The wildness that I had inherited while I was in Iraq, it was still in me when I got home. The sense of not caring. Not worried about anything."

His nightmares were intense. Alcohol was like medicine to calm his nerves, to help him forget. In the early days home, he tried cocaine, and says his coke habit got out of hand. Then, during a three-week summer training mission with his National Guard unit, he "detoxed" and did not touch coke again for years.

Then, for nine months, he went AWOL (absent without leave) from the National Guard and let his hair grow long. He was afraid if he stayed in the Army, he would be sent back to Iraq. Eventually a trio of sergeants came knocking on the door of his mother's house, where he was living.

They gave him a choice: Come with them and stay in the service – or get kicked out and receive a dishonorable discharge.

He went with them. They took him to get a haircut, then back to his unit, and he fell into place as if he had never missed a day. His drinking continued the entire time he was in the Army, even during weekend drills. He was sent home many times for being drunk on duty, but he was never punished. The military, he says, gave him a pass because of his PTSD.

As he had in Iraq, Cross tried to get help. VA doctors sent him to support groups that focused on anger management and substance abuse, but nothing ever stuck. He was not worried about his drinking; he thought he had his life under control.

There was even a point at which he did. In 2014, he had almost stopped drinking and was going to recovery groups three days a week at the VA. He enrolled in classes at RCC, looking to the future. Then things went off the rails again.

He asked a buddy from school, who was preparing a shot of heroin for himself, to shoot him up, too. Cross calls it the biggest mistake he has ever made. Soon, heroin created a monster he could not control, but he abandoned heroin when he discovered the painkiller Opana. From then on, he shot up pain pills.

"Before I got involved with drugs," he says, "the idea of using a needle, of shooting up heroin, that was all taboo to me. That was something so far out of reach that I couldn't believe that anybody could ever do something like that. I certainly thought that I would never do something like that."

He spent all his time and money on drugs – about $3,000 a month, which was most of his disability check, and sometimes more. If he didn't have cash for a fix, he borrowed it. On occasion, he "borrowed" it from relatives' wallets. Sometimes drug dealers gave him drugs on credit 'til payday.

Since he could not afford to live on his own, he lived with his mother. When she kicked him out, he lived with his dad. "Nobody wanted me to live with them," he says. "I was a drug addict."

His brother became his best drug buddy. Roger had enlisted a year before Preston but did not see duty in Iraq until a few years after his younger brother returned. Now they were battling the same demons.

Motivation to change

Cross does not paint a pretty picture of his life as an addict.

He had always thought a person on drugs could just stop, cold turkey, and move on. But he discovered it was not that easy. Every day, he woke up "dopesick," which is what drug users call the symptoms of withdrawal.

"I had to have that pain pill to feel normal again. If I didn't have money, I'd find money. I'd borrow money. It was a mission every day just to get money, just to feel normal. That was no life. Wake up, find money, feel normal."

He spent time in homeless shelters. He had run-ins with law enforcement. He was robbed numerous times, once at knifepoint. "I was with the people who had nothing, who had lost everything."

He checked himself into the hospital time after time. "I wanted to stop so bad I couldn't stand it. I could not find that code."

In the fall of 2018, he found the "code" – the motivation – while he was in a Virginia jail cell.

He and his girlfriend, Linsey, had been traveling on Interstate 77 near Wytheville, Virginia – on the way to visit her family in Kentucky – when the alternator on her car went out. It was close to midnight. They called for roadside assistance. Linsey went to a nearby gas station, and he waited with the car, calmly shooting up cocaine while he waited.

Cross did not know it was standard procedure for law enforcement to accompany tow truck drivers on such late-night calls. He was surprised when a deputy showed up, and even more surprised when the deputy, looking through a window, saw a syringe cap, giving him probable cause to search the vehicle, where he found a $20 bag of coke.

As Cross sat in jail, he envisioned the new life he wanted to build with Linsey falling apart. It was the motivation he needed to change. "You've got to have a purpose," he says.

"I just wanted that new life so bad. I finally had a girl, and I finally wanted that family, and I wanted that new life so bad that I made a decision, and I haven't turned back since."

When he returned home, he went to a clinic and got a prescription for Suboxone, a medication used to treat opioid addiction. He completed an intensive outpatient program. More than a year later, he is still drug-free.

Battling occasional urges to use can still be a struggle, Cross said, but it is getting easier. "I still think about it sometimes, but it's few and far between."

He attends support group meetings twice a week with what he calls his "battle buddies" in Salisbury: "We're all suffering from the same problems. We all have similar stories."

On his day in court in Virginia, he was sentenced to a year's probation and ordered to do 100 hours of community service.

'That wasn't me'

Cross cannot reconcile who he is today with the man he was during his active addiction.

"It's extremely hard to believe that was me," he says. "And people I grew up with can't believe that was me. … I look back on it and I think about all the people I hurt. My life that I had destroyed at that time. All the people that I have broken the trust with. I cannot believe that was me who done all that. I really can't. Because that isn't me, and everybody knew that wasn't me."

He says he used

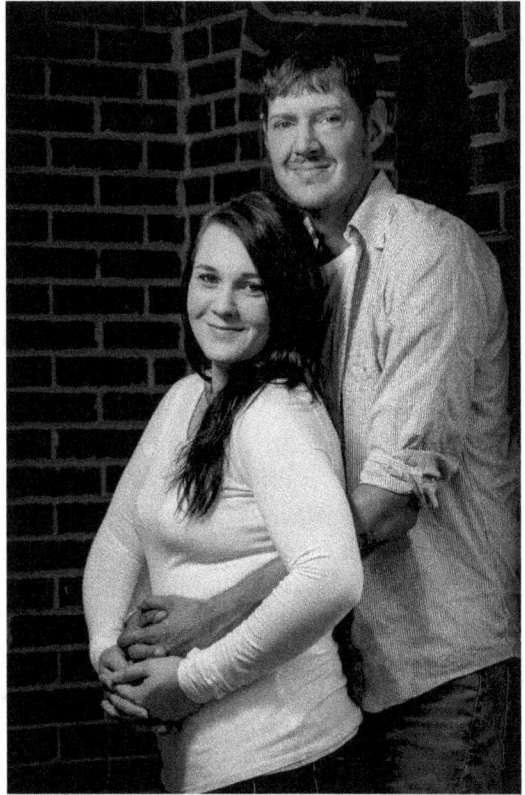

HIS REASON – Preston Cross credits his girlfriend, Linsey Draper, with giving him a reason to leave drugs behind. She is expecting their child, a girl, in March of 2020. (Contributed photo)

to look at people whose sole purpose seemed to be to get high and wonder why they did not just stop.

"What are y'all doin'? How could you live your life like that? How could you lose everything and still be OK and still do drugs? I couldn't understand why. I thought they could just, just fix your life, get better. But it was – it is not that easy."

His family thought quitting was easy, too.

"Now they realize what it took for me and my brother to get clean. It took an act of God for us to get clean."

His message to those with family still in addiction: "Don't give up on their loved ones that's struggling, to never give up on 'em, to always push them to want to get better, to want to get help."

Cross is proud that if someone asks how Preston is doing these days, his family has good things to say.

PICKING UP
THE PIECES

It got to the point I knew if one had died, I'd be burying the other.

In the family
Krista Childress and Sara Cross watched men they loved go down

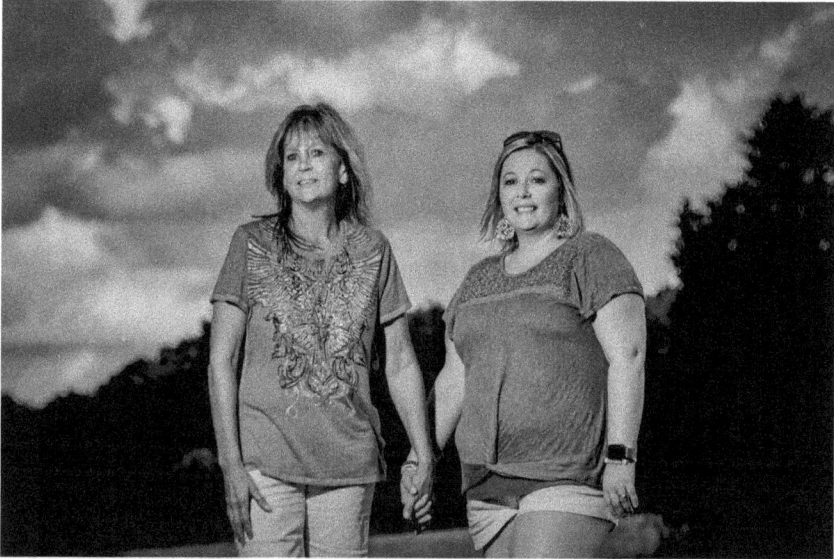

SOMEONE TO LEAN ON – Krista Childress, left, and her daughter-in-law, Sara Cross, helped each other through the dark days when Krista's sons, Roger and Preston, were in active addiction. Roger and Sara are married. (Photograph by Paul Church/Courtesy The Courier-Tribune)

Few things are worse than a mother whose child lives to do drugs. One of those things is having two children who will lie, scheme, manipulate, and steal to get the next pain pill or white powder to shoot up.

Krista Childress was in that place not long ago.

Her younger son, Preston Cross – home from the war in Iraq, a man who had lost most everything because he spent nearly every penny of his monthly disability check on drugs – was living in her basement. Each night she prayed that she would not wake up and find him dead in bed.

She was certain that her older son, Roger Cross, would not live long if Preston died from an overdose. Roger was home from the war in Iraq, too; he also devoted all his time and money to tracking down and doing drugs.

"It got to the point I knew if one had died," Childress says,

93

"I'd be burying the other."

Both men were in and out of detox and rehab many times. They usually returned to drugs as soon as they were "free" again.

Today, Childress no longer fears how her son's stories will end. Preston has been drug-free for a year; Roger just wrapped up six months in a treatment program in Texas. Both say they are changed men.

When Roger's mother and wife, Sara Cross, visited him in Texas over the summer, he told them he had written a name on a piece of paper that he carried in his shirt pocket. Over his heart. He told them he prays for the person.

"He needs somebody to love him and pray for him," Roger said, "just like y'all did for me."

The person? Roger's former drug dealer.

Drinking to forget

The Cross boys were born 11 months apart, Roger in February of 1985, Preston the following January.

They never caused trouble in school, or anywhere else, but school was not their thing. His senior year, Roger dropped out shortly after the birth of a son; then both his infant son and his son's mother died – tough territory for a teen to navigate. Preston, a junior, dropped out, too.

Both earned GEDs at Randolph Community College and entered the workaday world. After 9/11, Roger had decided that he was going to enlist someday. He joined the Army National Guard in 2004; Preston, who had dreamed of being in the Army since he was a kid, signed up a couple of years later. He chose the same specialty as his older brother, field artillery.

Preston was the first brother to set boots on the ground in the Middle East. He was there for 10 months in 2006 and 2007, manning a machine gun to protect military convoys crisscrossing the country. Roger and Sara met in March 2005 and wed in May. He deployed the day after they were married but did not head to Iraq until 2009.

Roger's job in Iraq was driving large trucks to transport military equipment. He and Sara kept in touch during his year's tour of duty via phone calls and Skype, but he never talked about anything bad. Neither brother talked about what they did or saw in Iraq, while they were there or after they came home.

Eventually, both were diagnosed with service-related post-traumatic stress disorder, or PTSD. Neither had been big drinkers before their service in a war zone; after, they both drank more.

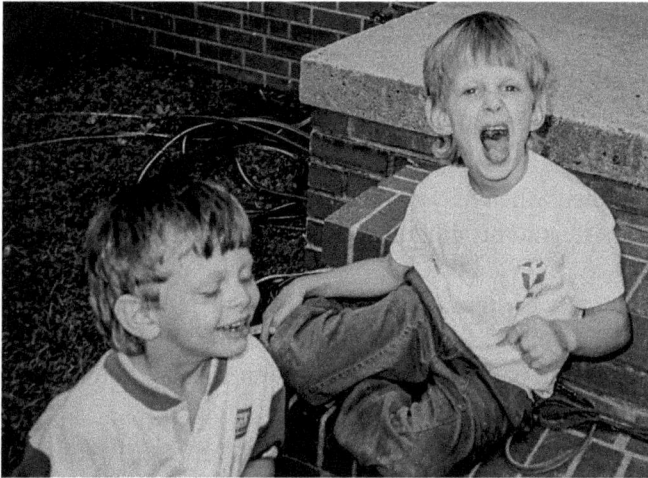

BEST BUDDIES – Roger (on the left in both pictures) and Preston Cross were born 11 months apart. Inseparable brothers, they both enlisted in the Army National Guard and served tours of durty in Iraq. (Contributed photos)

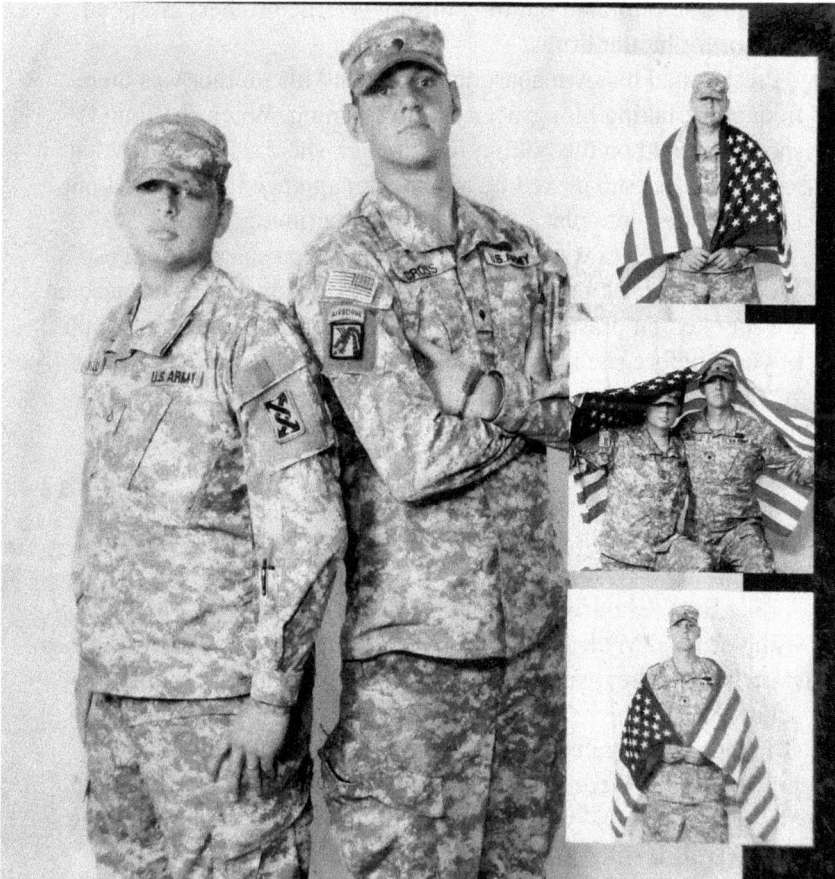

They drank to forget. They graduated to more powerful drugs and forgot more than the past. They forgot their families in the present.

His mother says the Preston who returned home was not the man who had left to serve his country. The new Preston drank from morning to night; he could not keep a job. "He was so scared of every single noise," she says. "He was paranoid."

Sometimes, when he was drinking, Preston talked about suicide. One night he told his mother that he did not want to remember anymore. Convinced that he was going to kill himself, she secured an involuntary commitment. When she visited the mental health facility where he was taken, Preston was in a stupor from drugs the doctors had ordered. The intervention was not helpful. It only made him mad at her.

After he came home, Roger returned to a good job, and for a while, was a dependable worker, a good provider for his family. On weekends, he hit the bottle hard.

Stronger stuff

Their lives spiraled out of control when the brothers swapped alcohol for harder drugs.

Preston had his own apartment then, and his mother was there frequently, taking him groceries and cleaning. When she found spoons burned on the bottom in a drawer, she did not know what to think. After she picked up a toboggan and needles tumbled out, the pieces fell into place. Preston was shooting up heroin.

For a time, Sara was in the dark about her husband's drug use. When he cut back on drinking, she did not know it was because he was hooked on prescription painkillers. He used pills for a couple of years before she knew it. The news was a shock.

"If you'd asked me when I met Roger," she says, "if he'd ever turn out to be somebody that was on drugs, I'd say, 'Not in a million years. Never.'"

Later, Roger injured his jaw in a workplace accident. Now he had a new source of painkillers to abuse – a prescription in his name.

Like Sara, Childress was shocked to know that her sons were using drugs: "My boys were raised in church. My daddy was a preacher … They were good kids. They never got in trouble in school."

Things deteriorated when the brothers started using drugs together. They were relentless in their quest and often stayed out all night. They also were in and out of detox and treatment at the W.G. (Bill) Hefner VA Medical Center in Salisbury.

They never went at the same time. One would say he was sick of doing drugs and check in for treatment. The next month, the other would promise to go the VA tomorrow – if he could have $50 to buy a pill today. Sara says such tactics worked because she was desperate for an answer.

"It was like I held onto any inkling of maybe him getting better because I knew that it was either going to come down to Roger was going to be dead; I was going to lose my kids; or me and Roger were just not going to be able to be together … And I would do almost anything to get him to somewhere where I thought they might could fix him."

Sometimes, Preston would stay in treatment for 30 days or more. Roger never lasted that long at the VA, but twice went to Camp Hope in Texas, a faith-based treatment program for combat veterans with PTSD. The first time, in 2016, he left after 51 days. The second time, in 2017, he skipped out after 21 days. He left on payday – the first day of the month when his government check is deposited in the bank. (Both brothers are on disability for PTSD.)

"They would get paid on the first," Childress says. "Well, by the third, they were broke. They went through their whole check. Well, that's when they would decide to go to detox. So, they would stay in detox until payday."

When one left detox, the other usually picked him up – and the merry-go-round continued.

"Even if one got clean," Childress says, "they'd always mess up when they got with the other one. They just fed off each other."

Stay away

When he started spending so much on drugs that he could not afford an apartment, Preston moved back into his mother's home.

One day she noticed a red, swollen place on his arm and asked about it. Preston told her he did not know what it was. He said he might have cut himself. He said he needed to go to VA, and then changed his mind. Maybe it will get better, he said. The next morning, he could barely sit up, his fever was sky high, and he was throwing up.

A medical procedure at the VA hospital to treat the place – which turned out to be infection from a needle – left a gaping hole in his arm. He told his mother that it was not his first infection from a needle. But he did not stop shooting up.

Sometimes Roger asked his mother to share the prescription

pain pills she takes for back problems. He feigned backaches, toothaches, headaches. Later, both boys begged for pills because they were sick and shaking. They were "dopesick" – experiencing withdrawal because they needed a fix. Before she wised up, Childress gave them pills. She was trying to help.

When she bought and moved into her family homeplace, Childress implored Preston not to use drugs in the house where her father, the preacher, and her mother had lived for 40 years. The enclosed carport had served as his pastor's study. "It's not sacred," she says, "but, to me, it was sacred because nothing like that's ever been in this house."

When she found spoons, syringes and other paraphernalia in his room, she kicked Preston out. Exhausted and losing weight from constant worry and sleepless nights, she took another step. She told both her boys to stay away: "I could not take no more. I could not do it no more. I was wiped out."

'Just getting normal'

Eventually, Roger could not keep a job. Sara worked to support the household, but usually Roger's disability check went to buy drugs. More than once, she asked relatives to help pay a power bill, buy groceries, or put gas in her car.

She found needles hidden in the house and learned that he was shooting up pills, an opioid pain medication named Opana. Later, whenever she found more hiding places and more needles, Roger had excuses: That was old. I haven't done that in months. Preston left that here.

"It was any excuse he could give me that he thought I would believe," she says. "And I knew, but he had a way, he had a way about him of making me think that he was actually telling the truth. But that's just the name of their game. Manipulation is just the name of the game when it comes to drugs.

"Even though I knew what was going on there was times I would turn around and be like, 'Well, maybe he's telling me the truth.' And I knew he wasn't. But I thought he might be."

Home was not a happy place. If his family was at home, Roger went out. If he was home, Sara and the kids stayed away. When they returned, she always made the children wait in the car while she checked inside. She did not know what she might find. Would Roger be alive?

Sara could not understand why Roger was destroying their lives. He tried to tell her: "He said that I'm not getting high anymore. I'm just getting normal."

Childress recalls Preston saying something similar: 'I've got to have it just so I can get up out of bed. I've got to have it just so I can carry on a conversation.'

When Roger tried to quit using drugs – and he tried many times – Sara shielded their children. She did not want them to see him shaking uncontrollably, throwing up, a shadow of himself.

But quitting was not something he could manage on his own.

During the worst days of his addiction, he took things from the house to swap or sell to fund his drug habit: the lawnmower, the TV, the children's Xbox, his daughter's cell phone, even the coffee pot. In those days, Sara slept with her wallet and car keys.

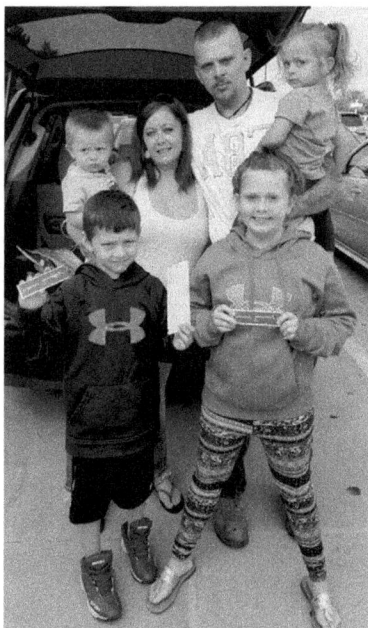

FAMILY OF SIX – Preston and Sara Cross have four children, clockwise from left, Liam, Layne, Lillie, and Londyn. Roger plans to have frank conversations with his children so they understand about bad choices he made which led to many undesirable things. (Contributed photo)

Pack and leave

Preston got clean a year ago by going to a Suboxone clinic. Roger also got a prescription of Suboxone but wound up trading his for other drugs.

After Preston stopped using, the brothers did not interact much, and Roger did not go out much. He holed up in a bedroom with the door locked, emerging only to get something to eat, to use the bathroom, or to go get more drugs.

Sara sometimes threatened to leave. The truth was she hoped that if someone moved out it would be Roger because she did not want to disrupt her children's lives any more.

Childress encouraged Sara to stick it out. She feared that Roger would go into a tailspin if left alone. Then, her thinking changed. Roger had never overdosed, never been arrested, never faced any negative consequences for his drug abuse. She thought it was time to change that and suggested that Sara pack, take the children, and leave.

One evening not long after that, Roger refused to spend any money for food. Sara knew he wanted the money for drugs. They argued, and he left. She was angry and tired of living under such stress and uncertainty. She told the children to pack

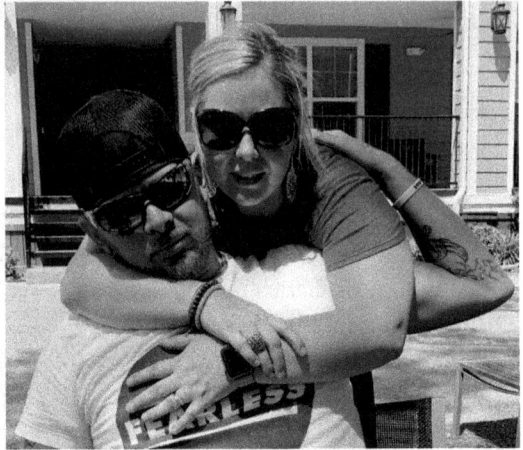
Roger and Sara Cross at Camp Hope in 2019.
(Contributed photo)

some clothes. Of course, they asked what was happening. She was crying so hard she could scarcely tell them.

Roger called that evening, March 8, 2019, and asked if she would bring him something to eat when she came home. She told him she was not coming home. He called daily, crying. "The best thing you can do is do what's best for you," Sara told him. "Get better. Get clean. You've got to care about yourself."

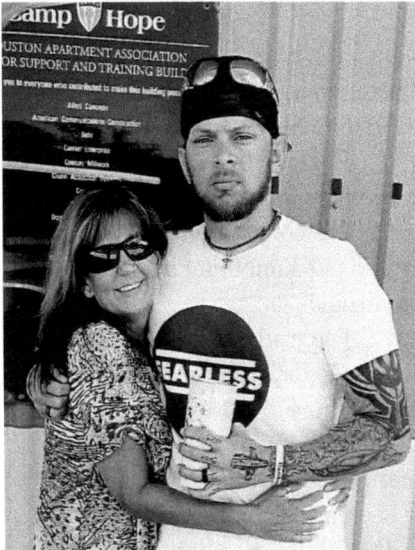
Roger and Krista at Camp Hope in 2019.
(Contributed photo)

Less than two weeks later, he had booked himself into the Texas program he had left two times before. He checked in on March 26. If she had not taken the children and left, he told her recently, he probably would still be doing drugs.

Roger has written his story as part of his recovery and told Sara that he wants to sit down and share it one day. She knows there likely will be much she does not know. What she knows is heartbreaking enough: "We lost houses. We lost cars. We lost so much: just time, memories with the kids, everything."

'Love an addict'

Sara knows the struggle is not over.

Roger has fence-building and heart-mending to do with his children, Lillie, who is 13, Layne, 10, Londyn, 6, and Liam, 4. He has started building those relationships by phone and says he is prepared to have frank conversations when he comes home so his children understand about his bad choices which led to so many undesirable things. He also says he knows that his actions consigned everyone in the family to their own PTSD. Healing will take time.

"For the first time in six years," Sara says, "I feel like things are coming together, and we're going to be able to be a family."

Childress is hopeful, too. "It's like, finally, for the first time in years, my boys can be brothers, instead of drug buddies."

She says she is thankful for the help her sons received to become clean and sober; she wonders about people who do not have such resources.

"There's addicts out there that don't have the help like our veterans do, you know, they've got to pay for it. There's no way my boys could have ever went through the treatment they have if we had to pay for it."

The women acknowledge that drug users make choices but push back against what some people believe – that addicts are worthless, individuals who deserve every terrible thing that comes their way, even dying of an overdose.

"Well, evidently it's not their son," Childress says. "Or their daughter."

"Or their husband," Sara adds. "Or the father of their kids."

Her husband and brother-in-law are great people with great hearts, Sara says, not the self-centered souls they appeared to be when they were in active addiction.

"You can't really judge an addict by what they did during active addiction," she says. "You can't do that. It's not fair to them, and it's not fair to beat yourself up over why somebody would treat you that way. That's not who they are at all.

"You should love an addict, and maybe you hate what they do, but you love them because nine times out of ten, if you see an addict, they want to be different. They don't want to be that person."

I look in my son's eyes, and he looks so lost.
Like he's a shell of the person that he was.

'He's my baby'
Melissa Huffman raised her son and now is raising his boys

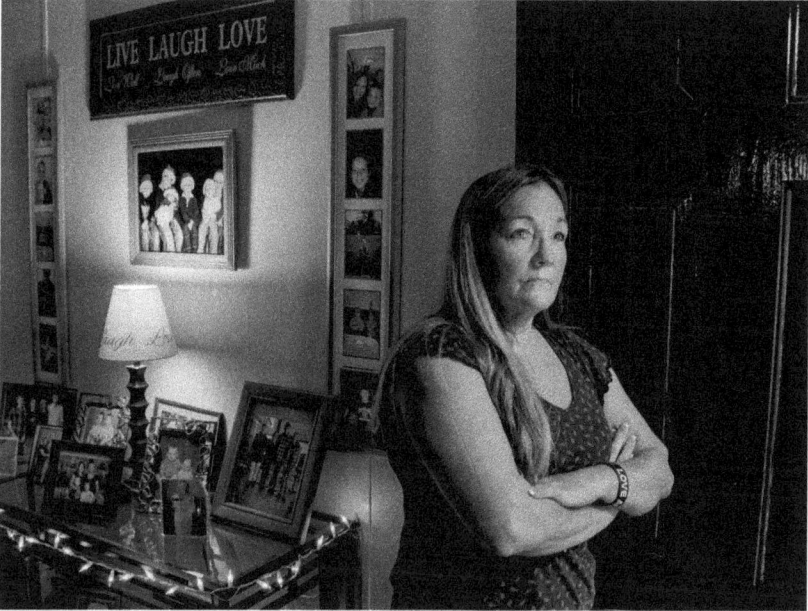

STEPPING UP – Melissa Huffman adopted her grandsons Jayden and Dalton after the court stripped her son, Mark Kellam, and his wife of their parental rights. She says many grandparents are raising their grandchildren due to substance abuse problems. (Photograph by Paul Church/Courtesy The Courier-Tribune)

Melissa Huffman is raising two of her son's children. They used to call her MawMaw. Now they call her Mom.

Jayden, who is 12, and Dalton, 11, have lived with Huffman for most of their lives, and she adopted them five years ago.

The primary reason Mark Kellam, who is Huffman's son, and Megan Pate lost custody of their boys is substance abuse, but neglect included a 4-year-old Jayden being attacked twice in two months by a dog in the home. The first time the dog nearly bit off one of his ears.

Shortly after that Social Services temporarily placed the brothers under Huffman's care to give Mark and Megan time to get their lives in order. The original order for six months was extended to a year, then two, as Mark and Megan failed drug tests or showed up high – or not at all – for scheduled visits with their children.

Finally, case workers recommended, and the court granted, termination of Mark and Megan's parental rights.

Recently, Huffman and Dalton were sitting at their kitchen table talking. She told him about someone who had died from a drug overdose.

"When we get that call that dad overdosed," he told her, "I'm going to feel a lot of sad feelings, but I'm going to feel a lot of really angry feelings, too."

He would be angry, he explained, because an overdose is something that can be prevented – by not doing drugs.

"And that's why I'm keeping them involved in awareness," Huffman says, "because I want them to know one bad choice can change their whole entire life. One."

'He looks so lost'

Kellam's drug of choice these days is methamphetamine. Over the years, his name has been in the newspaper law log often for drug possession, resisting arrest, not showing up in court, and other charges.

In the spring of 2019, he made the front page, under the headline: "Caroline's gone." Some northeastern Randolph County residents came home one Wednesday in April to find their garden hose flooding their driveway. Someone had rummaged in the garage; their dog was gone; and the dog's water bowl had been cleaned and filled with water.

A deputy responding to another call in the area, this one about a trespasser, spotted Kellam, who was carrying blankets and frozen food – things taken from the garage. He also had a dog.

He was charged with several felonies, including breaking and entering and larceny after breaking/entering, and served with outstanding warrants, one from Guilford County for simple assault, one from Randolph for resisting a public officer.

When he talked with his mother later, he told her that the dog did not have any water, so he broke into the dog lot and took care of that. Then he went into the garage. He told her he took the blankets and food because he thought the world was going to end.

"I look in my son's eyes, and he looks so lost," Huffman says. "Like he's a shell of the person that he was."

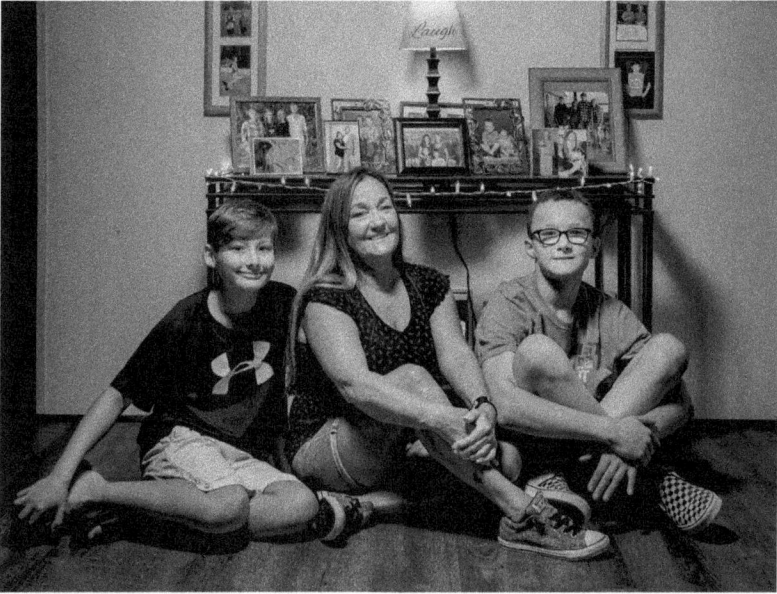

THEY CALL HER MOM – Grandsons Dalton, left, and Jayden flank Melissa Huffman in their home east of Asheboro. Jayden is on the A-B honor roll; Dalton makes all As. She says she quit smoking three years ago to stay as healthy as she can as they grow up. (Photo by Paul Church/Courtesy The Courier-Tribune)

Tears of joy

When Mark was born, Huffman cried. The doctor asked if she wanted a girl. She already had two daughters. She wanted a son with all her heart. They were tears of joy.

She and Mark's father separated when Mark was 9. It was not an easy time for a boy that age. As he grew, playing sports helped him forget his life off the field.

By high school, Mark's athletic talents were on display on the diamond, the field, and the mat: He played baseball. He was captain of the football team. He was a three-time state wrestling champ.

His wrestling coach – a hunting man with hunting dogs – once bragged about Mark: "I hate to compare it to a dog," the coach told Huffman, "but some dogs have it, and some dogs don't. Mark's got it."

He told her Mark was on track to earn a college scholarship to wrestle most anywhere he wanted to go. She remembers sitting in the bleachers on Friday nights under the lights in Charles R. Gregory Stadium, the home of the Randleman Tigers football team. She recalls hearing Mark's voice reverberate across the field as he fired up teammates in the huddle.

Then Mark started seeing a girl named Megan, and sports fell into second place. Huffman is sure they drank and smoked marijuana. She talked to her son about it. He told her he knew what he was doing. Harder drugs came later. She is not sure when.

"The coach told me, 'I can see him falling off. You're going to have to snatch him back,'" Huffman says. "I tell people it was like I woke up one morning, and he was so far out there that I just, I couldn't, I couldn't grab him back. It just happened so quickly."

Megan got pregnant. The couple's

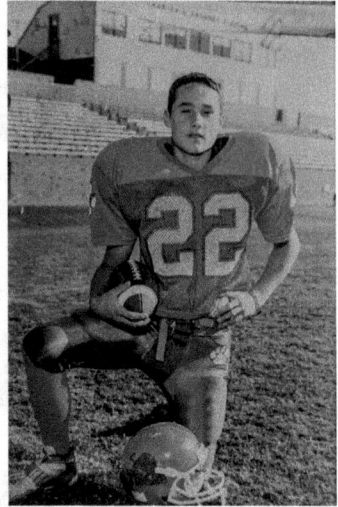

GLORY DAYS – Mark Kellam was a stellar athlete (captain of the football team and state champion wrestler) at Randleman High School. (Contributed photo)

first child was a baby they named Jayden; 360 days later, Dalton was born. Mark and Megan married after the boys were born. By then, Mark had dropped out of school and had a job in construction.

They lived with his grandmother at first, but later got a place of their own. Huffman remembers getting calls about parties or fights at their house. "You might want to go check on the boys," the caller – a friend or a neighbor – would say.

When Jayden and Dalton first came to live with her, she could not take them shopping: They ran amok. They were not bad kids; they just did not know any better. Today Jayden is on the A-B honor roll; Dalton makes all As.

'This drug is powerful'

About a year ago, Mark called his mother, crying and frantic, and asked her to pick him up. Someone, he said, was going to kill him.

"Have you ever seen someone really geeked out on meth?" Huffman asks. "It's very scary."

That night was the first time she had ever seen Mark strung out. He got into her car and explained that someone with chain saws and knives had lined a bathtub with plastic and planned to chop his body to pieces.

She was terrified, but tried to stay calm, hoping she could

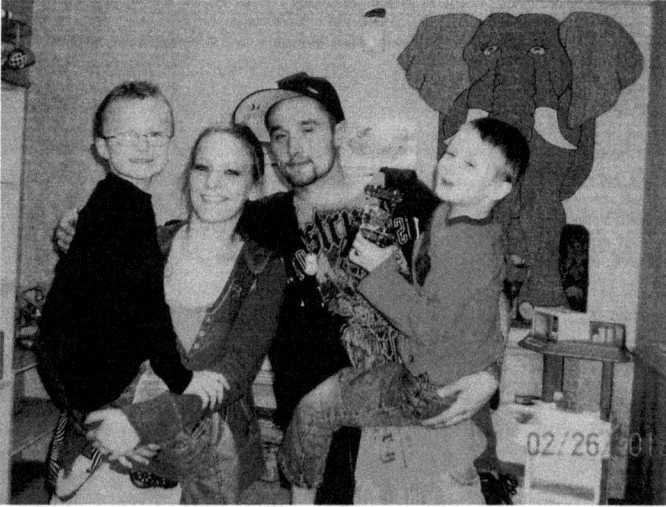

DAYS GONE BY – Mark Kellam and his wife Megan smile for the camera with Jayden, left, and Dalton. (Contributed photo)

calm him. She asked if he wanted to go to police. He didn't. She headed toward his grandmother's house, where he lives; she was not going to take him to her house to be around the boys.

Suddenly, he started looking at his hands, screaming: "Oh, my God, oh, my God, I know what they did."

"What did they do?" she asked.

"They put the gun in my hand, and now the residue's on me, and they're going to say that I killed him."

She tried to soothe his fears by telling Mark that if somebody died, investigators would be able to determine time of death. She told him she would vouch for his whereabouts: "I've got your back," she said.

When they got to his grandmother's house he would not get out of the car. He thought there were people in the trees, watching.

One time, Mark called police and reported that there were people in a wooded area in north Asheboro who wanted to kill him. He told the officer who responded to slam him to the ground and pretend to arrest him, so he could get away. The officer called for backup. They took him to the hospital, where he bit a security guard and had to be strapped to the bed.

Huffman said that one time when Mark showed up at her house "out of his head," she called 911 and asked for an ambulance to take him to a hospital. Law enforcement showed up first. Mark ran. "I ended up sitting in the yard," she says, "listening to dogs chase my son."

Mark has been in and out of therapy. He has "graduated" from two treatment programs, and he has been kicked out of a treatment program. The last time he went was 4.5 years ago. Today, he tells his mom he does not need help.

"This drug is powerful," Huffman says. "It's nothing like this world has ever seen."

'Six little eyes'

Recently Mark wrote on Facebook that he was looking for work. He said he is good with art and construction, pretty much anything with his hands, and that he is not lazy or looking for a handout.

He wrote that all he ever wanted to do was to stand on his own two feet, but there was nothing to stand on. He said all he needs to better himself is a shot. Please consider that I might not be what everyone says, he wrote. He added that he was not asking for selfish reasons – that he had six little eyes that do not know who their father really is.

Huffman says the social media post breaks her heart. The "six little eyes" are Jayden, Dalton, and a younger brother who is in the care of his great-grandparents.

"He's talking about six little eyes that he wants to make proud. He gets in these moods sometimes," she says. "He's said several things lately, you can tell he's thinking, but it doesn't go much past that."

Huffman says Mark and Megan, their mother, cannot visit the boys while they are in active addiction. "I adopted them to protect them, and I'm not going to let anything interfere with that."

The two are still married but no longer together. He has not seen the boys in months; she has not seen them in years. Huffman has issued invitations to both her son and daughter-in-law: Come live with me, help with the boys, and I'll help you. Neither has accepted.

Once, after several months in rehab, Mark came to his mom's house when he got out. He stayed two or three days and then called his "drug buddies" to come pick him up. Earlier this year, she says, her son was drug-free after spending 4.5 months in jail. When he was released, he did not call her – or his boys.

An addict's mom

Huffman is not immune to negative things people say about those in addiction. Sometimes those people make her angry, and sometimes they make her sad, but she knows they do not understand.

"I don't wish this on my worst enemy," she says. "I hope that this never happens to your child. If it does happen to your child, you will change your attitude in a minute."

It's simple, she says: She does not condone her son's drug use, but she loves him.

Whenever she sees a first responder, she stops to thank him (or her). She asks to shake hands. She says she understands they may be sick and tired of overdose calls – of trying to save people who are not trying to save themselves. And she says, "Thank you."

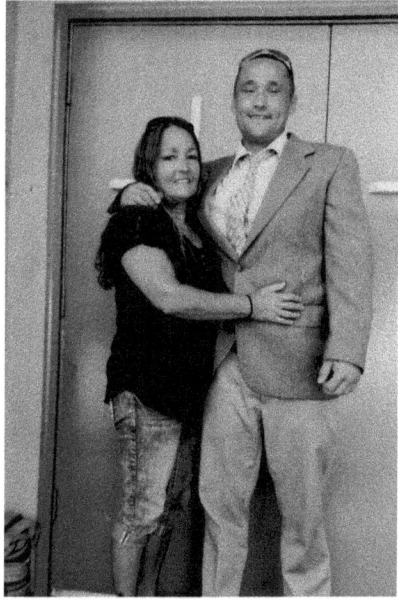

A REASON TO SMILE – Melissa Huffman and her son, Mark Kellam, pose during a happier time, when he was drug-free. (Contributed photo)

"There are a lot of us mothers that would say the same thing to you," she adds. "And every time you go out on an overdose call, and you save someone, you are saving someone's child, someone's mother, someone's father, someone's sister, or someone's brother."

She takes medications for anxiety and depression; she has sought mental health counseling and joined support groups. One is an online group called The Addict's Mom. Huffman says it has more than 25,000 members.

"Every day, there are, I would say, four to eight moms who are losing their children, who have gotten that call. It's a very sad, hard life to live. … The heart of an addict's mom is the most broken-hearted you will ever see. I grieve my son even though he's still alive."

'He's my baby'

Mark tells his mother that he does drugs to get out of his head. He also tells her: "I'm OK, even when I'm not OK, Ma."

Several friends have lost children to overdose.

"I've been to so many funerals, and especially within the last two years, it's pitiful. A lot of my son's friends have died. In my head, I've got his funeral planned out. I know that sounds terrible. I go to bed every single night, thinking, this is the night. Or every single day, I think, you know, this is the day."

She says she is at peace, knowing that her son has a strong faith, a relationship with Jesus, and that she has done everything she knows to do to help him. She says he knows that she loves him. And she knows that he loves her.

"My son is gone already," she says. "I'm just waiting for the call, the official call, but my son is already gone -- the son that I knew is gone. And I know, there's hope, where there's breath, there's hope, but sometimes, after so long, you start to lose hope, and it's heartbreaking.

"... I'd give anything to help him. If love could fix him, he'd have been fixed a long time ago. I mean, he's my baby. He's grown, but he's my baby."

RESOURCES
FOR HELP

SUBSTANCE ABUSE ASSESSMENT/TREATMENT

For immediate treatment help in North Carolina,
call 1-800-610-4673.
www.treatment-centers.net/directory/north-carolina
Mobile Crisis Unit/Therapeutic Alternatives 1-877-626-1772
Asheboro 336-626-1700
Randleman 336-495-2700

DETOX

• **Novant Health Forsyth Medical Center**, Winston Salem, N.C., 336-718-5000. Accepts men and women with Medicaid, private insurance or self-pay.

• **Old Vineyard Behavioral Health**, Winston Salem, N.C., 336-794-3550. Accepts, men and women with Medicaid, private insurance or self-pay. www.oldvineyardbhs.com.

• **Addiction Recovery Care Association (ARCA)**, 336-784-9470. Accepts men and women for detox. Cannot have active Medicaid or private insurance to detox at ARCA; they have county funding for detox. www.arcanc.org.

• **Solus Christus**, East Bend, N.C., 336-813-3007. Accepts women only. A safe house while waiting for a rehab to open up. www.soluschristusinc.org.

RESIDENTIAL AND OUTPATIENT

• **Evans-Blount Total Access Care**, 525 White Oak St., Asheboro, N.C., 704-886-1934. Accepts uninsured patients. Email: mjohnson@evansblounttac.com.

• **Ready 4 Change**, Asheboro, N.C., and Greensboro, N.C., 336-907-7819.

• **Daymark Recovery**, Asheboro, 336-633-7000; Archdale, 336-431-0700; Lexington, 336-242-2450; High Point, 336-899-1550. www.daymarkrecovery org.

• **Randolph Fellowship Homes**, Asheboro, N.C., 336-625-1637. Houses for men and women. www.randolphrecovery.com .

• **TASC (Treatment Accountability for Safer Communities)** through Insight Human Services, 336-725-8389; help@ insightnc.org; www.insightnc.org/intervention/tasc.

• **TROSA (Triangle Residential Options for Substance**

Abusers Inc.); 1820 James St., Durham, N.C., 919-419-1059. www.trosainc.org.

• **A Path of Hope**, 1675 E. Center St. Ext., Lexington, N.C., 336-248-8914; email: pathofhope@apathofhope.org; www. apathofhope.org.

• **Robert S. Swain Recovery Center**, 932 Old U.S. Hwy. 70, Black Mountain, N.C., 828-338-2162. www.insightnc.org.

• **Naaman's Recovery Village**, High Point, N.C., 336-410-5098. A 12-to-18-month residential recovery program. There is no fee. Currently accepts men only. Contact Pastor Jack Martin. naamansrecoveryvillage.org.

• **Pierced Ministries and Rehab Inc.** – Archdale, NC - A 9-to-12-month residential recovery program for men and women. The entry fee is $750; in some ases the entry fee may be waived or paid after the program is complete. Contact Ronnie Meindl, 336-337-5817. www.pierced4me.org.

• **Bethel Colony of Mercy**, Lenoir, N.C., 828-754-3781. A 62-day residential recovery program for men only. The entry fee is $250. www.bethelcolony.org.

• **Addiction Recovery Care Association (ARCA)**, Winston Salem, N.C., 336-784-9470. A residential treatment facility for men and women. Accepts Medicaid; does not accept private insurance; also has county funding. www.arcanc.org.

• **WISH (Women and Infants Services for Health)**, 725 North Highland Ave., Winston-Salem, N.C., 336-397-7500. This program allows women with children to go to treatment with children and live with them. Accepts Medicaid; if clients do not have Medicaid, it's free. They do not provide detox; detox has to be done elsewhere before transter to their facility.

• **Mary's House**, 520 Guilford Ave., Greensboro, N.C., 336-275-0820. Permanent housing in High Point and Greensboro and intensive inpatient provided at Greensboro location only. Allows mothers to bring children; can have up to eight families in the program at a time.

• **Healing Transitions**, 1251 Goode St., Raleigh, N.C., 919-838-9800. Inpatient, outpatient and overnight emergency shelter and family services and detox. No cost to clients. 117 beds.

• **Caring Services Inc (CSI)**, 102 Chestnut Drive High Point, N.C., 336-886-5549. www.caringservices.org.

• **High Point Regional**, High Point, N.C., 336-878-6000. Detox, residential, day treatment, IOP. Some indigent, major insurance, Medicaid, Medicare.

- **DART – Cherry**, Goldsboro, N.C., 888-788-4660. 90-day residential authorized by probation.
- **Black Mountain**, 828-669-4174. 90-day residential. Authorized by probation.
- **ADATC-Butner**, 919-575-7000.
- **Walter B. Jones**, Greenville, N.C., 252-830-3426.
- **First at Blue Ridge**, Ridgecrest, N.C., 828-669-0011.
- **Samaritan Colony**, Rockingham, N.C., 910-895-3243.
- **House of Prayer**, Jamestown, N.C., 336-882-1026.
- **Living Free Ministries**, Snow Camp, N.C., 336-376-5066.
- **Will's Place**, Albemarle, N.C., 980-581-8001.
- **Teen Challenge**, Greensboro, N.C., 336-292-7795.
- **Pinehurst Treatment Centers**, Pinehurst, N.C., 910-24-3669.
- **First Step Services**, multiple locations, 919-833-8899.
- **Therapeutic Alternatives/Mobile Crisis**, 962 S. Fayetteville St., Asheboro, N.C., 877-626-1772. Email: courteney.schenck@ mytahome.com.
- **Triad Therapy Mental Health Center LLC**, 131 Davis St., Suite N, Asheboro, N.C., 336-896-0904. Email: Info@ triadtherapy.com.
- **Guilford County Alcohol and Drug Services (ADS)**, 301 E. Washington St., Suite 101, Greensboro, N.C., 336-333-6860. Email: counselor@adsyes.org.
- **Bright Heart Health**, 1150 Revolution Mill Drive, Greensboro, N.C., 919-230-1232. Email: jciampi@ brighthearthealth.com.
- **Cross Roads Treatment Centers**, 2706 North Church St., Greensboro, N.C., 336-272-9990.
- **Caring Services**, 102 Chestnut Drive, High Point, N.C., 336-886-5594. Email: info@caringservices.org.
- **Evans-Blount Total Access Care**, 2031 Martin Luther King Jr. Drive, Greensboro, N.C., 336-271-5888. Email: mjohnson@ evansblounttac.com.
- **Fellowship Hall**, 5140 Dunstan Road, Greensboro, N.C., 800-659-3381. Email: infofellowship@fellowshiphall.org.
- **High Point Behavioral Health**, 601 N. Elm St., High Point, N.C., 800-525-9375.
- **Presbyterian Counseling Center**, 3713 Richfield Road, Greensboro, N.C., 336-288-1484. Email: jsweet.pcc@gmail.com.
- **Ringer Center**, 213 E. Bessemer Ave., Greensboro, N.C., 336-379-7146. Email: ringercenter@aol.com.

- **Triad Behavioral Resources**, 810 Warren St., Greensboro, N.C., 336-389-1413.
- **Triad Psychiatric and Counseling Center**, 603 Dolley Madison Road, Suite 100, Greensboro, N.C., 336-632-3505.
- **Wesley Long Hospital**, 2400 W. Friendly Ave., Greensboro, N.C., 336-832-9615.
- **"A" Assessment and Counseling Center**, 127 Worth St. Asheboro, N.C., 336-918-0213. DWI assessments and counseling.
- **Alcohol & Drug Services**, 842 E. Pritchard St., Asheboro, 336-633-7257 (Asheboro office); 336-333-6860 (Greensboro office). www.adsyes.org.
- **Randolph Health Internal Medicine – Suboxone Clinic**, 237A N. Fayetteville St., Asheboro, N.C., 336-625-3248.
- **Triad Therapy**, 131B Davis St., Asheboro office, 336-629-7774; Winston-Salem office, 336-896-0994.
- **Carolina Counseling Assoc.**, Asheboro, 336-629-4471. Outpatient mental health and substance abuse individual. Medicaid.

HOUSING/SHELTERS
- **Shelter of Hope**, 133 W. Wainman Ave., Asheboro, N.C., 336-318-0012. For men only.
- **Family Crisis Center**, 624 S. Fayetteville St., Asheboro, N.C., 336-629-4159. For victims of domestic (women and children).

EMERGENCY SERVICES
- **Randolph County Department of Social Services**, Asheboro, N.C., 336-683-8000.
- **Christians United Outreach Center (CUOC)**, 135 Sunset Ave., Asheboro, N.C., 336-625-1500.
- **Randolph County Sheriff's Office**, 727 McDowell Road, Asheboro, N.C., 336-318-6699.
- **Asheboro Police Department**, 205 E. Academy St., Asheboro, N.C., 336-626-1300.
- **Archdale Police Department**, 305 Balfour Drive, Archdale, N.C., 336-434-3134.

MEDICAL SERVICES
- **Randolph Health**, 364 White Oak St., Asheboro, N.C., 336-625-5151.
- **High Point Regional Hospital**, 601 N. Elm St., High Point, N.C., 336-878-6000.

• **Randolph County Health Department**, 2222 S. Fayetteville St., Asheboro, N.C. Call 336-318-6882 about AIDS informatiion, communicable diseases, dental health, family planning, immunization, and WIC.

• **Randolph Family Health Care/Sexually Transmitted Disease Hotline**, 800-227-8922, 1831 N. Fayetteville St., Asheboro, N.C., 336-672-1300.

• **Your Choice Pregnancy Care Center**, 530 S. Cox St., Asheboro, N.C., 336-629-9988 or 1-800-395-4357.

• **RAPE (24-hour crisis line)**, 336-629-4159.

• **Randolph Health Community Health Services**, 336-629-8896, ext. 5214.

HARM REDUCTION

Upon release from jail, detox, rehab, hospital stay, or any amount of time in recovery, be aware that tolerance is lower, and it is easy to overdose if you choose to use at this time. DO NOT go back to a previous dose, and DO NOT use alone. Have someone with you who can administer Narcan/naloxone.

Once a person has overdosed and was revived, he or she is more apt to overdose again. It lowers tolerance each time, and it becomes easier to overdose and lead to a fatal overdose.

• **Community Paramedic Program/EMS and Health Department**, Kendall Phillips, 336-318-6197.

• **Community Hope Alliance**, 1406 N. Fayetteville St., Unit L, Asheboro, N.C., Kelly Link, 336-465-1431; Ashley Hedrick, 336-633-8974. Naloxone access, mobile syringe exchange, community outreach/awareness, and more.

• **GCSTOP (Guilford County Solution to the Opioid Problem),** Greensboro, N.C., Chase Holleman, 336-505-8122. Naloxone access, syringe exchange, peer support, fentanyl test strips, and more.

• **Twin City Harm Reduction**, Winston-Salem, N.C., 336-705-9881. Syringe access, naloxone access, Hep C testing, counseling, and more.

• **Urban Survivors Union**, Greensboro, N.C., 1116 Grove St., Greensboro N.C., 336-669-5543. Syringe access, naloxone access, fentanyl test strips, peer support, and more.

* **Senate Bill 794, effective 2016, authorizes organizations to establish and operate Syringe Exchange Programs,** which gives limited immunity to employees, volunteers and participants.

* **According to NC-GS-90-113.22, effective 2016, participants of a Syringe Exchange Program are granted immunity from prosecution for carrying syringes** and other injection equipment.

* **HB850 "Tell Law Officer" law, effective 2013, always disclose you have a syringe before it is found in a search;** doing so grants immunity from paraphernalia charges.

* **"911 Good Samaritan Law"; North Carolina protects people who ask for help from 911, the police or EMS because they or another person is overdosing.** People cannot be tried in court for having small amounts of drugs or paraphernalia. They also cannot get in trouble with probation or parole. You must give your name to 911 or to EMS or police that come.

* **The law also covers people who administer naloxone/ Narcan to a person thought to be overdosing, even if they were not.** If you suspect an overdose, it's safer to give the reversal medication. It does no harm to a person if it turns out it was not an overdose.

* **Never abandon a friend, or even a stranger, who is overdosing.** Call 911. Administer naloxone as directed, if available. Give rescue breathing: Tilt head back, pinch nose, and blow one hard breath into mouth every five seconds. If person is still unresponsive after two minutes, give another dose and continue rescue breathing until EMS arrives. If naloxone is not available, perform rescue breathing until help arrives, but call 911 first.

* **Please note that Hep C and/or AIDS cannot be contracted from mouth to mouth**, even if saliva enters your mouth. It is contracted through blood. If overdose victim is bleeding from the mouth, proceed with caution. But please don't let someone die because you are afraid of contracting a communicable disease; it is highly unlikely.

www.ingramcontent.com/pod-product-compliance
Lightning Source LLC
Chambersburg PA
CBHW050736030426
42336CB00012B/1590